The Bird Flu Handbook: What is Asian Influenza and What We Need To Know To Be Prepared for a Pandemic?

Written and Compiled by Manoj Kunda and Ward Lin

Published by Vayu Publishing
Copyright © 2005 Vayu Publishing

ISBN: 1-4116-5899-X

www.vayupublishing.com

Cover Art:

NCP 1603 - Emergency hospital during influenza epidemic,
Camp Funston, Kansas.

Reeve 15183 - U.S. Army Field Hospital No. 29, Hollerich,
Luxembourg, Interior View - Influenza Ward.

Armed Forces Institute of Pathology, National Museum of
Health and Medicine

TABLE OF CONTENTS

CHAPTER ONE

WHAT IS INFLUENZA?

This chapter will provide an introduction into Influenza, and some of the symptoms and treatments associated with it. Since Bird Flu (Avian Influenza) is a form of Influenza that has the potential to cross over from animals into humans, it is important to gain an understanding of the broader scope of the virus.

Influenza

Overview

Influenza is caused by a virus that attacks mainly the upper respiratory tract – the nose, throat and bronchi and rarely also the lungs. The infection usually lasts for about a week. It is characterized by sudden onset of high fever, myalgia, headache and severe malaise, non-productive cough, sore throat, and rhinitis. Most people recover within one to two weeks without requiring any medical treatment. In the very young, the elderly and people suffering from medical conditions such as lung diseases, diabetes, cancer, kidney or heart problems, influenza poses a serious risk. In these people, the infection may lead to severe complications of underlying diseases, pneumonia and death.

Influenza rapidly spreads around the world in seasonal epidemics and imposes a considerable economic burden in the form of hospital and other health care costs and lost productivity.

In annual influenza epidemics, 5-15% of the population are affected with upper respiratory tract infections. Hospitalization and deaths mainly occur in high-risk groups (elderly, chronically ill). Although difficult to assess, these annual epidemics are thought to result in between three and five million cases of severe illness and between

250,000 and 500,000 deaths every year around the world. Most deaths currently associated with influenza in industrialized countries occur among the elderly over 65 years of age.

Much less is known about the impact of influenza in the developing world. However, influenza outbreaks in the tropics where viral transmission normally continues year-round tend to have high attack and case-fatality rates. For example, during an influenza outbreak in Madagascar in 2002, more than 27,000 cases were reported within three months and 800 deaths occurred despite rapid intervention. An investigation of this outbreak, coordinated by the World Health Organization (WHO), found that there were severe health consequences in poorly nourished populations with limited access to adequate health care (see "Outbreak of influenza, Madagascar, July-August 2002," Weekly Epidemiological Record). It is not possible to extrapolate the exact annual burden of influenza in the tropics from data from such occasional and severe outbreaks.

The Virus

The currently circulating influenza viruses that cause human disease are divided into two groups: A and B. Influenza A has 2 subtypes which are important for humans: A(H3N2) and A(H1N1), of which the former is currently associated with most deaths. Influenza viruses are defined by 2 different protein components, known as antigens, on the surface of the virus. They are spike-like features called haemagglutinin (H) and neuraminidase (N) components.

The genetic makeup of influenza viruses allows frequent minor genetic changes, known as antigenic drift, and these changes require annual reformulation of influenza vaccines.

Pandemic Influenza

Three times in the last century, the influenza A viruses have undergone major genetic changes mainly in their H-component, resulting in global pandemics and large tolls in terms of both disease and deaths. The most infamous pandemic was "Spanish Flu" which affected large parts of the world population and is thought to have killed at least 40 million people in 1918-1919. More recently, two other influenza A pandemics occurred in 1957 ("Asian influenza") and 1968 ("Hong Kong influenza") and caused significant morbidity and mortality globally. In contrast to current influenza epidemics, these pandemics were associated with severe outcomes also among healthy younger persons, albeit not on such a dramatic scale as the "Spanish flu" where the death rate was highest among healthy young adults.

Most recently, limited outbreaks of a new influenza subtype A(H5N1) directly transmitted from birds to humans have occurred in Hong Kong Special Administrative Region of China in 1997 and 2003.

Transmission

The virus is easily passed from person to person through the air by droplets and small particles excreted when infected individuals cough or sneeze. The influenza virus enters the body through the nose or throat. It then takes between one and four days for the person to develop symptoms. Someone suffering from influenza can be infectious from the day before they develop symptoms until seven days afterwards.

Disease spreads very quickly among the population especially in crowded circumstances. Cold and dry weather enables the virus to survive longer outside the body than in other conditions and, as a consequence, seasonal epidemics in temperate areas appear in winter.

Diagnosis

Respiratory illness caused by influenza is difficult to distinguish from illness caused by other respiratory pathogens on the basis of symptoms alone. However, during laboratory-confirmed influenza outbreaks, the majority of persons seeking medical advice for upper respiratory tract infections are likely to be infected by influenza. Laboratory confirmation will be required between annual influenza epidemics. Rapid diagnostic tests have recently become available that can be used to detect influenza viruses within 30 minutes.

Despite the availability of rapid diagnostic tests, the collection of clinical specimens for viral culture remains critical to provide information regarding circulating influenza subtypes and strains. This is needed to guide decisions regarding influenza treatment and chemoprophylaxis and to formulate vaccine for the coming year.

Prevention: Influenza Vaccines

Vaccination is the principal measure for preventing influenza and reducing the impact of epidemics. Various types of influenza vaccines have been available and used for more than 60 years. They are safe and effective in preventing both mild and severe outcomes of influenza (see WHO position paper, "Influenza vaccines", Weekly Epidemiological Record).

It is recommended that elderly persons, and persons of any age who are considered at "high risk" for influenza-related complications due to underlying health conditions, should be vaccinated. Among the elderly, vaccination is thought to reduce influenza-related morbidity by 60% and influenza-related mortality by 70-80%. Among healthy adults the vaccine is very effective (70-90%) in terms of reducing influenza morbidity, and vaccination has been shown to have substantial health-related and economic benefits in this age group. The effectiveness of influenza vaccine depends primarily on the age and immunocompetence of the vaccine recipient and the degree of similarity between the viruses in the vaccine and those in circulation. Influenza vaccination can reduce both health-care costs and productivity losses associated with influenza illness. (see "Recommendations for the use of inactivated influenza vaccines and other preventive measures," Weekly Epidemiological Record).

All current inactivated influenza vaccines contain trace levels of egg protein and should not be used by individuals with egg protein allergies.

Constant genetic changes in influenza viruses mean that the vaccines' virus composition must be adjusted annually to include the most recent circulating influenza A(H3N2), A(H1N1) and influenza B viruses.

The WHO's Global Influenza Surveillance Network writes the annual vaccine recipe. The network, a partnership of 112 National Influenza Centres in 83 countries, is responsible for monitoring the influenza viruses circulating in humans and rapidly identifying new strains. Based on information collected by the Network, WHO recommends annually a vaccine that targets the 3 most virulent strains in circulation.

Treatment and Prophylaxis: Antiviral Agents

For most people influenza is an upper respiratory tract infection that lasts several days and requires symptomatic treatment only. Within days, the person's body will eliminate the virus. Antibiotics, such as penicillin, which are designed to kill bacteria, cannot attack the virus. Therefore antibiotics have no role in treating influenza in otherwise healthy people although they are used to treat complications.

Antiviral drugs for influenza are an important adjunct to influenza vaccine for the treatment and prevention of influenza. However, they are not a substitute for vaccination. For several years, four antiviral drugs that act by preventing influenza virus replication have been available. They differ in terms of their pharmacokinetics, side effects, routes of administration, target age groups, dosages, and costs.

When taken before infection or during early stage of the disease (within two days of illness onset), antivirals may help prevent infection, and if infection has already taken hold, their early administration may reduce the duration of symptoms by one to two days.

For several years, amantadine and rimantadine were the only antiviral drugs. However, whilst relatively inexpensive, these drugs are effective only against type A influenza, and may be associated with severe adverse effects (including delirium and seizures that occur mostly in elderly persons on higher doses). When used for prophylaxis of pandemic influenza at lower doses, such adverse events are far less likely. In addition, the virus tends to develop resistance to these drugs.

A new class of antivirals, the neuraminidase inhibitors, has been developed. Such drugs, zanamivir and oseltamivir, have fewer adverse side effects (although zanamivir may exacerbate asthma or other chronic lung diseases) and the virus less often develops resistance . However, these drugs are expensive and currently not available for use in many countries.

In severe influenza, admission to hospital, intensive care, antibiotic therapy to prevent secondary infection and breathing support may be required.

Note: The source material for this chapter was obtained from the World Health Organization website.

CHAPTER TWO

WHAT IS BIRD FLU (AVIAN INFLUENZA)?

Avian Influenza

Avian influenza is an infectious disease of birds caused by type A strains of the influenza virus. The disease, which was first identified in Italy more than 100 years ago, occurs worldwide.

All birds are thought to be susceptible to infection with avian influenza, though some species are more resistant to infection than others. Infection causes a wide spectrum of symptoms in birds, ranging from mild illness to a highly contagious and rapidly fatal disease resulting in severe epidemics. The latter is known as "highly pathogenic avian influenza". This form is characterized by sudden onset, severe illness, and rapid death, with a mortality that can approach 100%.

Fifteen subtypes of influenza virus are known to infect birds, thus providing an extensive reservoir of influenza viruses potentially circulating in bird populations. To date, all outbreaks of the highly pathogenic form have been caused by influenza A viruses of subtypes H5 and H7.

Migratory waterfowl – most notably wild ducks – are the natural reservoir of avian influenza viruses, and these birds are also the most resistant to infection. Domestic poultry, including chickens and turkeys, are particularly susceptible to epidemics of rapidly fatal influenza.

Direct or indirect contact of domestic flocks with wild migratory waterfowl has been implicated as a frequent cause of epidemics. Live bird markets have also played an important role in the spread of epidemics.

Recent research has shown that viruses of low pathogenicity can, after circulation for sometimes short periods in a poultry population, mutate into highly pathogenic viruses. During a 1983–1984 epidemic in the United States of America, the H5N2 virus initially caused low mortality, but within six months became highly pathogenic, with a mortality approaching 90%. Control of the outbreak required destruction of more than 17 million birds at a cost of nearly US$ 65 million. During a 1999–2001 epidemic in Italy, the H7N1 virus, initially of low pathogenicity, mutated within 9 months to a highly pathogenic form. More than 13 million birds died or were destroyed.

The quarantining of infected farms and destruction of infected or potentially exposed flocks are standard control measures aimed at preventing spread to other farms and eventual establishment of the virus in a country's poultry population. Apart from being highly contagious, avian influenza viruses are readily transmitted from farm to farm by mechanical means, such as by contaminated equipment, vehicles, feed, cages, or clothing. Highly pathogenic viruses can survive for long periods in the environment, especially when temperatures are low. Stringent sanitary measures on farms can, however, confer some degree of protection.

In the absence of prompt control measures backed by good surveillance, epidemics can last for years. For example, an epidemic of H5N2 avian influenza, which began in Mexico in 1992, started with low pathogenicity, evolved to the highly fatal form, and was not controlled until 1995.

A Constantly Mutating Virus: Two Consequences

All type A influenza viruses, including those that regularly cause seasonal epidemics of influenza in humans, are genetically labile and well adapted to elude host defenses. Influenza viruses lack mechanisms for the "proofreading" and repair of errors that occur during replication. As a result of these uncorrected errors, the genetic composition of the viruses changes as they replicate in humans and animals, and the existing strain is replaced with a new antigenic variant. These constant, permanent and usually small changes in the antigenic composition of influenza A viruses are known as antigenic "drift".

The tendency of influenza viruses to undergo frequent and permanent antigenic changes necessitates constant monitoring of the global influenza situation and annual adjustments in the composition of influenza vaccines. Both activities have been a cornerstone of the WHO Global Influenza Programme since its inception in 1947.

Influenza viruses have a second characteristic of great public health concern: influenza A viruses, including subtypes from different species, can swap or "reassort" genetic materials and merge. This reassortment process, known as antigenic "shift", results in a novel subtype different from both parent viruses. As populations will have no immunity to the new subtype, and as no existing vaccines can confer protection, antigenic shift has historically resulted in highly lethal pandemics. For this to happen, the novel subtype needs to have genes from human influenza viruses that make it readily transmissible from person to person for a sustainable period.

Conditions favourable for the emergence of antigenic shift have long been thought to involve humans living in close proximity to domestic poultry and pigs. Because pigs are susceptible to infection with both avian and mammalian viruses, including human strains, they can serve as a "mixing vessel" for the scrambling of genetic material from human and avian viruses, resulting in the emergence of a novel subtype. Recent events, however, have identified a second possible mechanism. Evidence is mounting that, for at least some of the 15 avian influenza virus subtypes circulating in bird populations, humans themselves can serve as the "mixing vessel".

Human Infection with Avian Influenza

Avian influenza viruses do not normally infect species other than birds and pigs. The first documented infection of humans with an avian influenza virus occurred in Hong Kong in 1997, when the H5N1 strain caused severe respiratory disease in 18 humans, of whom 6 died. The infection of humans coincided with an epidemic of highly pathogenic avian influenza, caused by the same strain, in Hong Kong's poultry population.

Extensive investigation of that outbreak determined that close contact with live infected poultry was the source of human infection. Studies at the genetic level further determined that the virus had jumped directly from birds to humans. Limited transmission to health care workers occurred, but did not cause severe disease.

Rapid destruction – within three days – of Hong Kong's entire poultry population, estimated at around 1.5 million birds, reduced opportunities for further direct transmission to humans, and may have averted a pandemic.

That event alarmed public health authorities, as it marked the first time that an avian influenza virus was transmitted directly to humans and caused severe illness with high mortality. Alarm mounted again in February 2003, when an outbreak of H5N1 avian influenza in Hong Kong caused 2 cases and 1 death in members of a family who had recently travelled to southern China. Another child in the family died during that visit, but the cause of death is not known.

Two other avian influenza viruses have recently caused illness in humans. An outbreak of highly pathogenic H7N7 avian influenza, which began in the Netherlands in February 2003, caused the death of one veterinarian two months later, and mild illness in 83 other humans. Mild cases of avian influenza H9N2 in children occurred in Hong Kong in 1999 (two cases) and in mid-December 2003 (one case). H9N2 is not highly pathogenic in birds.

The most recent cause for alarm occurred in January 2004, when laboratory tests confirmed the presence of H5N1 influenza virus in human cases of severe respiratory disease in the northern part of Vietnam.

Why H5N1 is of Particular Concern

Of the 15 avian influenza virus subtypes, H5N1 is of particular concern for several reasons. H5N1 mutates rapidly and has a documented propensity to acquire genes from viruses infecting other animal species. Its ability to cause severe disease in humans has now been documented on two occasions. In addition, laboratory studies have demonstrated that isolates from this virus have a high pathogenicity and can cause severe disease in humans. Birds that survive infection excrete virus for at least 10 days, orally and in faeces, thus facilitating further spread at live poultry markets and by migratory birds.

The epidemic of highly pathogenic avian influenza caused by H5N1, which began in mid-December 2003 in the Republic of Korea and is now being seen in other Asian countries, is therefore of particular public health concern. H5N1 variants demonstrated a capacity to directly infect humans in 1997, and have done so again in Viet Nam in January 2004. The spread of infection in birds increases the opportunities for direct infection of humans. If more humans become infected over time, the likelihood also increases that humans, if concurrently infected with human and avian influenza strains, could serve as the "mixing vessel" for the emergence of a novel subtype with sufficient human genes to be easily transmitted from person to person. Such an event would mark the start of an influenza pandemic.

Influenza Pandemics: an they be averted?

Based on historical patterns, influenza pandemics can be expected to occur, on average, three to four times each century when new virus subtypes emerge and are readily transmitted from person to person. However, the occurrence of influenza pandemics is unpredictable. In the 20th century, the great influenza pandemic of 1918–1919, which caused an estimated 40 to 50 million deaths worldwide, was followed by pandemics in 1957–1958 and 1968–1969.

Experts agree that another influenza pandemic is inevitable and possibly imminent.

Most influenza experts also agree that the prompt culling of Hong Kong's entire poultry population in 1997 probably averted a pandemic.

Several measures can help minimize the global public health risks that could arise from large outbreaks of highly pathogenic H5N1 avian influenza in birds. An immediate priority is to halt further spread of epidemics in poultry populations. This strategy works to reduce opportunities for human exposure to the virus. Vaccination of persons at high risk of exposure to infected poultry, using existing vaccines effective against currently circulating human influenza strains, can reduce the likelihood of co-infection of humans with avian and influenza strains, and thus reduce the risk that genes will be exchanged. Workers involved in the culling of poultry flocks must be protected, by proper clothing and equipment, against infection. These workers should also receive antiviral drugs as a prophylactic measure.

When cases of avian influenza in humans occur, information on the extent of influenza infection in animals as well as humans and on circulating influenza viruses is urgently needed to aid the assessment of risks to public health and to guide the best protective measures. Thorough investigation of each case is also essential. While WHO and the members of its global influenza network, together with other international agencies, can assist with many of these activities, the successful containment of public health risks also depends on the epidemiological and laboratory capacity of affected countries and the adequacy of surveillance systems already in place.

While all these activities can reduce the likelihood that a pandemic strain will emerge, the question of whether another influenza pandemic can be averted cannot be answered with certainty.

Treatment of human cases of H5N1 Avian Influenza

Published information about the clinical course of human infection with H5N1 avian influenza is limited to studies of cases in the 1997 Hong Kong outbreak. In that outbreak, patients developed symptoms of fever, sore throat, cough and, in several of the fatal cases, severe respiratory distress secondary to viral pneumonia. Previously healthy adults and children, and some with chronic medical conditions, were affected.

Tests for diagnosing all influenza strains of animals and humans are rapid and reliable. Many laboratories in the WHO global influenza network have the necessary high-security facilities and reagents for performing these tests as well as considerable experience. Rapid bedside tests for the diagnosis of human influenza are also available, but do not have the precision of the more extensive laboratory testing that is currently needed to fully understand the most recent cases and determine whether human infection is spreading, either directly from birds or from person to person.

Antiviral drugs, some of which can be used for both treatment and prevention, are clinically effective against influenza A virus strains in otherwise healthy adults and children, but have some limitations. Some of these drugs are also expensive and supplies are limited.

Experience in the production of influenza vaccines is also considerable, particularly as vaccine composition changes each year to match changes in circulating virus due to antigenic drift. However, at least four months would be needed to produce a new vaccine, in significant quantities, capable of conferring protection against a new virus subtype.

Note: The source material for this chapter was obtained from the World Health Organization website.

CHAPTER THREE

WHAT IS AN INFLUENZA PANDEMIC, AND WHY SHOULD WE BE AFRAID?

Pandemic: A Worldwide Outbreak of Influenza

An influenza pandemic is a global outbreak of disease that occurs when a new influenza A virus appears or "emerges" in the human population, causes serious illness, and then spreads easily from person to person worldwide. Pandemics are different from seasonal outbreaks or "epidemics" of influenza. Seasonal outbreaks are caused by subtypes of influenza viruses that already circulate among people, whereas pandemic outbreaks are caused by new subtypes, by subtypes that have never circulated among people, or by subtypes that have not circulated among people for a long time. Past influenza pandemics have led to high levels of illness, death, social disruption, and economic loss.

Appearance (Emergence) of Pandemic Influenza Viruses

There are many different subtypes of Influenza or "flu" viruses. The subtypes differ based upon certain proteins on the surface of the virus (the hemagglutinin or "HA" protein and the neuraminidase or the "NA" protein).

Pandemic viruses emerge as a result of a process called "antigenic shift," which causes an abrupt or sudden, major change in influenza A viruses. These changes are caused by new combinations of the HA and/or NA proteins on the surface of the virus. Changes results in a new influenza A virus subtype. The appearance of a new influenza A virus subtype is the first step toward a pandemic; however, to cause a pandemic, the new virus subtype also must have the capacity to spread easily from person to person. Once a new pandemic influenza virus emerges and spreads, it usually becomes established among people and moves around or "circulates" for many years as seasonal epidemics of influenza. The U.S. Centers for Disease Control and Prevention (CDC) and the World Health Organization (WHO) have large surveillance programs to monitor and detect influenza activity around the world, including the emergence of possible pandemic strains of influenza virus.

Influenza Pandemics During the 20th Century

During the 20th century, the emergence of several new influenza A virus subtypes caused three pandemics, all of which spread around the world within a year of being detected.

- 1918-19, "Spanish flu," [A (H1N1)], caused the highest number of known influenza deaths. (However, the actual influenza virus subtype was not detected in the 1918-19 pandemic). More than 500,000 people died in the United States, and up to 50 million people may have died worldwide. Many people died within the first few days after infection, and others died of secondary complications. Nearly half of those who died were young, healthy adults. Influenza A (H1N1) viruses still circulate today after being introduced again into the human population in 1977.

- 1957-58, "Asian flu," [A (H2N2)], caused about 70,000 deaths in the United States. First identified in China in late February 1957, the Asian flu spread to the United States by June 1957.

- 1968-69, " Hong Kong flu," [A (H3N2)], caused about 34,000 deaths in the United States. This virus was first detected in Hong Kong in early 1968 and spread to the United States later that year. Influenza A (H3N2) viruses still circulate today.

Both the 1957-58 and 1968-69 pandemics were caused by viruses containing a combination of genes from a human influenza virus and an avian influenza virus. The 1918-19 pandemic virus appears to have an avian origin.

Stages of a Pandemic

WHO has developed a global influenza preparedness plan, which defines the stages of a pandemic, outlines the role of WHO, and makes recommendations for national measures before and during a pandemic. The phases are:

Interpandemic period

Phase 1: No new influenza virus subtypes have been detected in humans. An influenza virus subtype that has caused human infection may be present in animals. If present in animals, the risk of human infection or disease is considered to be low.

Phase 2: No new influenza virus subtypes have been detected in humans. However, a circulating animal influenza virus subtype poses a substantial risk of human disease.

Pandemic alert period

Phase 3: Human infection(s) with a new subtype, but no human-to-human spread, or at most rare instances of spread to a close contact.

Phase 4: Small cluster(s) with limited human-to-human transmission but spread is highly localized, suggesting that the virus is not well adapted to humans.

Phase 5: Larger cluster(s) but human-to-human spread still localized, suggesting that the virus is becoming increasingly better adapted to humans but may not yet be fully transmissible (substantial pandemic risk).

Pandemic period

Phase 6: Pandemic: increased and sustained transmission in general population.

Notes: The distinction between **phases 1** and **2** is based on the risk of human infection or disease resulting from circulating strains in animals. The distinction is based on various factors and their relative importance according to current scientific knowledge. Factors may include pathogenicity in animals and humans, occurrence in domesticated animals and livestock or only in wildlife, whether the virus is enzootic or epizootic, geographically localized or widespread, and other scientific parameters.

The distinction among **phases 3 , 4,** and **5** is based on an assessment of the risk of a pandemic. Various factors and their relative importance according to current scientific knowledge may be considered. Factors may include rate of transmission, geographical location and spread, severity of illness, presence of genes from human strains (if derived from an animal strain), and other scientific parameters.

Vaccines to Protect Against Pandemic Influenza Viruses

A vaccine probably would not be available in the early stages of a pandemic. When a new vaccine against an influenza virus is being developed, scientists around the world work together to select the virus strain that will offer the best protection against that virus. Manufacturers then use the selected strain to develop a vaccine. Once a potential pandemic strain of influenza virus is identified, it takes several months before a vaccine will be widely available. If a pandemic occurs, the U.S. government will work with many partner groups to make recommendations guiding the early use of available vaccine.

Antiviral Medications to Prevent and Treat Pandemic Influenza

Four different influenza antiviral medications (amantadine, rimantadine, oseltamivir, and zanamivir) are approved by the U.S. Food and Drug Administration (FDA) for the treatment and/or prevention of influenza. All four usually work against influenza A viruses. However, the drugs may not always work, because influenza virus strains can become resistant to one or more of these medications. For example, the influenza A (H5N1) viruses identified in human in Asia in 2004 and 2005 have been resistant to amantadine and rimantadine. Monitoring of avian viruses for resistance to influenza antiviral medications continues.

Preparing for the Next Pandemic

Many scientists believe it is only a matter of time until the next influenza pandemic occurs. The severity of the next pandemic cannot be predicted, but modeling studies suggest that the impact of a pandemic on the United States could be substantial. In the absence of any control measures (vaccination or drugs), it has been estimated that in the United States a "medium–level" pandemic could cause 89,000 to 207,000 deaths, 314,000 and 734,000 hospitalizations, 18 to 42 million outpatient visits, and another 20 to 47 million people being sick. Between 15% and 35% of the U.S. population could be affected by an influenza pandemic, and the economic impact could range between $71.3 and $166.5 billion.

Influenza pandemics are different from many of the threats for which public health and health-care systems are currently planning:

- A pandemic will last much longer than most public health emergencies and may include "waves" of influenza activity separated by months (in 20th century pandemics, a second wave of influenza activity occurred 3 to 12 months after the first wave).

- The numbers of health-care workers and first responders available to work can be expected to be reduced. They will be at high risk of illness through exposure in the community and in health-care settings, and some may have to miss work to care for ill family members.

- Resources in many locations could be limited, depending on the severity and spread of an influenza pandemic.

Because of these differences and the expected size of an influenza pandemic, it is important to plan preparedness activities that will permit a prompt and effective public health response. The U.S. Department of Health and Human Services (HHS) supports pandemic influenza activities in the areas of surveillance (detection), vaccine development and production, strategic stockpiling of antiviral medications, research, and risk communications. In May 2005, the U.S. Secretary of HHS created a multi-agency National Influenza Pandemic Preparedness and Response Task Group. This unified initiative involves CDC and many other agencies (international, national, state, local and private) in planning for a potential pandemic. Its responsibility includes revision of a U.S. National Pandemic Influenza Response and Preparedness Plan.

Note: The source material for this chapter was obtained from the Centers for Disease Control and Prevention website.

CHAPTER FOUR

HAVE THERE BEEN ANY PANDEMICS IN THE 20TH CENTURY?

Pandemics and Pandemic Scares in the 20th Century

Historical Overview

History suggests that influenza pandemics have probably happened during at least the last four centuries. During the 20th century, three pandemics and several "pandemic scares" occurred. These are described in more detail below.

1918: Spanish Flu

The Spanish Influenza pandemic is the catastrophe against which all modern pandemics are measured. It is estimated that approximately 20 to 40 percent of the worldwide population became ill and that over 20 million people died. Between September 1918 and April 1919, approximately 500,000 deaths from the flu occurred in the U.S. alone. Many people died from this very quickly. Some people who felt well in the morning became sick by noon, and were dead by nightfall. Those who did not succumb to the disease within the first few days often died of complications from the flu (such as pneumonia) caused by bacteria.

One of the most unusual aspects of the Spanish flu was its ability to kill young adults. The reasons for this remain uncertain. With the Spanish flu, mortality rates were high among healthy adults as well as the usual high-risk groups. The attack rate and mortality was highest among adults 20 to 50 years old. The severity of that virus has not been seen again.

1957: Asian Flu

In February 1957, the Asian influenza pandemic was first identified in the Far East. Immunity to this strain was rare in people less than 65 years of age, and a pandemic was predicted. In preparation, vaccine production began in late May 1957, and health officials increased surveillance for flu outbreaks.

Unlike the virus that caused the 1918 pandemic, the 1957 pandemic virus was quickly identified, due to advances in scientific technology. Vaccine was available in limited supply by August 1957. The virus came to the U.S. quietly, with a series of small outbreaks over the summer of 1957. When U.S. children went back to school in the fall, they spread the disease in classrooms and brought it home to their families. Infection rates were highest among school children, young adults, and pregnant women in October 1957. Most influenza-and pneumonia-related deaths occurred between September 1957 and March 1958. The elderly had the highest rates of death.

By December 1957, the worst seemed to be over. However, during January and February 1958, there was another wave of illness among the elderly. This is an example of the potential "second wave" of infections that can develop during a pandemic. The disease infects one group of people first, infections appear to decrease and then infections increase in a different part of the population. Although the Asian flu pandemic was not as devastating as the Spanish flu, about 69,800 people in the U.S. died.

1968: Hong Kong Flu

In early 1968, the Hong Kong influenza pandemic was first detected in Hong Kong. The first cases in the U.S. were detected as early as September of that year, but illness did not become widespread in the U.S. until December. Deaths from this virus peaked in December 1968 and January 1969. Those over the age of 65 were most likely to die. The same virus returned in 1970 and 1972. The number of deaths between September 1968 and March 1969 for this pandemic was 33,800, making it the mildest pandemic in the 20th century.

There could be several reasons why fewer people in the U.S. died due to this virus. First, the Hong Kong flu virus was similar in some ways to the Asian flu virus that circulated between 1957 and 1968. Earlier infections by the Asian flu virus might have provided some immunity against the Hong Kong flu virus that may have helped to reduce the severity of illness during the Hong Kong pandemic. Second, instead of peaking in September or October, like pandemic influenza had in the previous two pandemics, this pandemic did not gain momentum until near the school holidays in December. Since children were at home and did not infect one another at school, the rate of influenza illness among schoolchildren and their families declined. Third, improved medical care and antibiotics that are more effective for secondary bacterial infections were available for those who became ill.

1976: Swine Flu Scare

When a novel virus was first identified at Fort Dix, it was labeled the "killer flu." Experts were extremely concerned because the virus was thought to be related to the Spanish flu virus of 1918. The concern that a major pandemic could sweep across the world led to a mass vaccination campaign in the United States. In fact, the virus--later named "swine flu"--never moved outside the Fort Dix area. Research on the virus later showed that if it had spread, it would probably have been much less deadly than the Spanish flu.

1977: Russian Flu Scare

In May 1977, influenza A/H1N1 viruses isolated in northern China, spread rapidly, and caused epidemic disease in children and young adults (< 23 years) worldwide. The 1977 virus was similar to other A/H1N1 viruses that had circulated prior to 1957. (In 1957, the A/H1N1 virus was replaced by the new A/H2N2 viruses). Because of the timing of the appearance of these viruses, persons born before

1957 were likely to have been exposed to A/H1N1 viruses and to have developed immunity against A/H1N1 viruses. Therefore, when the A/H1N1 reappeared in 1977, many people over the age of 23 had some protection against the virus and it was primarily younger people who became ill from A/H1N1 infections. By January 1978, the virus had spread around the world, including the United States. Because illness occurred primarily in children, this event was not considered a true pandemic. Vaccine containing this virus was not produced in time for the 1977-78 season, but the virus was included in the 1978-79 vaccine.

1997: Avian Flu Scare

The most recent pandemic "scares" occurred in 1997 and 1999. In 1997, at least a few hundred people became infected with the avian A/H5N1 flu virus in Hong Kong and 18 people were hospitalized. Six of the hospitalized persons died. This virus was different because it moved directly from chickens to people, rather than having been altered by infecting pigs as an intermediate host. In addition, many of the most severe illnesses occurred in young adults similar to illnesses caused by the 1918 Spanish flu virus. To prevent the spread of this virus, all chickens (approximately 1.5 million) in Hong Kong were slaughtered. The avian flu did not easily spread from one person to another, and after the poultry slaughter, no new human infections were found.

In 1999, another novel avian flu virus – A/H9N2 – was found that caused illnesses in two children in Hong Kong. Although both of these viruses have not gone on to start pandemics, their continued presence in birds, their ability to infect humans, and the ability of influenza viruses to change and become more transmissible among people is an ongoing concern.

Note: The source material for this chapter was obtained from the United States Department of Health and Human Services website.

CHAPTER FIVE

TEN THINGS YOU NEED TO KNOW ABOUT PANDEMIC INFLUENZA

1. Pandemic Influenza is Different from Avian Influenza.

Avian influenza refers to a large group of different influenza viruses that primarily affect birds. On rare occasions, these bird viruses can infect other species, including pigs and humans. The vast majority of avian influenza viruses do not infect humans. An influenza pandemic happens when a new subtype emerges that has not previously circulated in humans.

For this reason, avian H5N1 is a strain with pandemic potential, since it might ultimately adapt into a strain that is contagious among humans. Once this adaptation occurs, it will no longer be a bird virus--it will be a human influenza virus. Influenza pandemics are caused by new influenza viruses that have adapted to humans.

2. Influenza Pandemics are Recurring Events.

An influenza pandemic is a rare but recurrent event. Three pandemics occurred in the previous century: "Spanish influenza" in 1918, "Asian influenza" in 1957, and "Hong Kong influenza" in 1968. The 1918 pandemic killed an estimated 40–50 million people worldwide. That pandemic, which was exceptional, is considered one of the deadliest disease events in human history. Subsequent pandemics were much milder, with an estimated 2 million deaths in 1957 and 1 million deaths in 1968.

A pandemic occurs when a new influenza virus emerges and starts spreading as easily as normal influenza – by coughing and sneezing. Because the virus is new, the human immune system will have no pre-existing immunity. This makes it likely that people who contract pandemic influenza will experience more serious disease than that caused by normal influenza.

3. The World may be on the Brink of Another Pandemic.

Health experts have been monitoring a new and extremely severe influenza virus – the H5N1 strain – for almost eight years. The H5N1 strain first infected humans in Hong Kong in 1997, causing 18 cases, including six deaths. Since mid-2003, this virus has caused the largest and most severe outbreaks in poultry on record. In December 2003, infections in people exposed to sick birds were identified.

Since then, over 100 human cases have been laboratory confirmed in four Asian countries (Cambodia, Indonesia, Thailand, and Viet Nam), and more than half of these people have died. Most cases have occurred in previously healthy children and young adults. Fortunately, the virus does not jump easily from birds to humans or spread readily and sustainably among humans. Should H5N1 evolve to a form as contagious as normal influenza, a pandemic could begin.

4. All Countries will be Affected.

Once a fully contagious virus emerges, its global spread is considered inevitable. Countries might, through measures such as border closures and travel restrictions, delay arrival of the virus, but cannot stop it. The pandemics of the previous century encircled the globe in 6 to 9 months, even when most international travel was by ship. Given the speed and volume of international air travel today, the virus could spread more rapidly, possibly reaching all continents in less than 3 months.

5. Widespread Illness will Occur.

Because most people will have no immunity to the pandemic virus, infection and illness rates are expected to be higher than during seasonal epidemics of normal influenza. Current projections for the next pandemic estimate that a substantial percentage of the world's population will require some form of medical care. Few countries have the staff, facilities, equipment, and hospital beds needed to cope with large numbers of people who suddenly fall ill.

6. Medical Supplies will be Inadequate.

Supplies of vaccines and antiviral drugs – the two most important medical interventions for reducing illness and deaths during a pandemic – will be inadequate in all countries at the start of a pandemic and for many months thereafter. Inadequate supplies of vaccines are of particular concern, as vaccines are considered the first line of defence for protecting populations. On present trends, many developing countries will have no access to vaccines throughout the duration of a pandemic.

7. Large Numbers of Deaths will Occur.

Historically, the number of deaths during a pandemic has varied greatly. Death rates are largely determined by four factors: the number of people who become infected, the virulence of the virus, the underlying characteristics and vulnerability of affected populations, and the effectiveness of preventive measures. Accurate predictions of mortality cannot be made before the pandemic virus emerges and begins to spread. All estimates of the number of deaths are purely speculative.

WHO has used a relatively conservative estimate – from 2 million to 7.4 million deaths – because it provides a useful and plausible planning target. This estimate is based on the comparatively mild 1957 pandemic. Estimates based on a more virulent virus, closer to the one seen in 1918, have been made and are much higher. However, the 1918 pandemic was considered exceptional.

8. Economic and Social Disruption will be Great.

High rates of illness and worker absenteeism are expected, and these will contribute to social and economic disruption. Past pandemics have spread globally in two and sometimes three waves. Not all parts of the world or of a single country are expected to be severely affected at the same time. Social and economic disruptions could be temporary, but may be amplified in today's closely interrelated and interdependent systems of trade and commerce. Social disruption may be greatest when rates of absenteeism impair essential services, such as power, transportation, and communications.

9. Every Country must be Prepared.

WHO has issued a series of recommended strategic actions for responding to the influenza pandemic threat. The actions are designed to provide different layers of defence that reflect the complexity of the evolving situation. Recommended actions are different for the present phase of pandemic alert, the emergence of a pandemic virus, and the declaration of a pandemic and its subsequent international spread.

10. WHO will Alert the World when the Pandemic Threat Increases.

WHO works closely with ministries of health and various public health organizations to support countries' surveillance of circulating influenza strains. A sensitive surveillance system that can detect emerging influenza strains is essential for the rapid detection of a pandemic virus.

Six distinct phases have been defined to facilitate pandemic preparedness planning, with roles defined for governments, industry, and WHO. The present situation is categorized as phase 3: a virus new to humans is causing infections, but does not spread easily from one person to another.

Note: The source material for this chapter was obtained from the World Health Organization website

CHAPTER SIX

ANSWERS TO YOUR MOST COMMON QUESTIONS ABOUT BIRD FLU (AVIAN INFLUENZA)

1) What is Avian Influenza?

Avian influenza, or "bird flu", is a contagious disease of animals caused by viruses that normally infect only birds and, less commonly, pigs. Avian influenza viruses are highly species-specific, but have, on rare occasions, crossed the species barrier to infect humans.

In domestic poultry, infection with avian influenza viruses causes two main forms of disease, distinguished by low and high extremes of virulence. The so-called "low pathogenic" form commonly causes only mild symptoms (ruffled feathers, a drop in egg production) and may easily go undetected. The highly pathogenic form is far more dramatic. It spreads very rapidly through poultry flocks, causes disease affecting multiple internal organs, and has a mortality that can approach 100%, often within 48 hours.

2) Which Viruses Cause Highly Pathogenic Disease?

Influenza A viruses[1] have 16 H subtypes and 9 N subtypes[2]. Only viruses of the H5 and H7 subtypes are known to cause the highly pathogenic form of the disease. However, not all viruses of the H5 and H7 subtypes are highly pathogenic and not all will cause severe disease in poultry.

On present understanding, H5 and H7 viruses are introduced to poultry flocks in their low pathogenic form. When allowed to circulate in poultry populations, the viruses can mutate, usually within a few months, into the highly pathogenic form. This is why the presence of an H5 or H7 virus in poultry is always cause for concern, even when the initial signs of infection are mild.

3) How are Bird Flu Viruses Different from Human Flu Viruses?

There are many different subtypes of type A influenza viruses. These subtypes differ because of certain proteins on the surface of the influenza A virus (hemagglutinin [HA] and neuraminidase [NA] proteins). There are 16 different HA subtypes and 9 different NA subtypes of flu A viruses. Many different combinations of HA and NA proteins are possible. Each combination is a different subtype. All known subtypes of flu A viruses can be found in birds. However, when we talk about "bird flu" viruses, we are referring to influenza A subtypes chiefly found in birds. They do not usually infect humans, even though we know they can. When we talk about "human flu viruses" we are referring to those subtypes that occur widely in humans. There are only three known A subtypes of human flu viruses (H1N1, H1N2, and H3N2); it is likely that some genetic parts of current human influenza A viruses came from birds originally. Influenza A viruses are constantly changing, and they might adapt over time to infect and spread among humans.

4) How is the Disease Spread?

Avian influenza is primarily spread by direct contact between healthy birds and infected birds, and through indirect contact with contaminated equipment and materials. The virus is excreted through the feces of infected birds and through secretions from the nose, mouth and eyes.

Contact with infected fecal material is the most common of bird-to-bird transmission. Wild ducks often introduce low pathogencicity into domestic flocks raised on range or in open flight pens through fecal contamination. Within a poultry house, transfer of the high pathogenicity avian influenza (HPAI) virus between birds can also occur via airborne secretions. The spread of avian influenza between poultry premises almost always follows the movement of contaminated people and equipment. Avian influenza also can be found on the outer surfaces of egg shells. Transfer of eggs is a potential means of avian influenza transmission. Airborne transmission of virus from farm to farm is highly unlikely under usual circumstances.

5) Do Migratory Birds Spread Highly Pathogenic Avian Influenza Viruses?

The role of migratory birds in the spread of highly pathogenic avian influenza is not fully understood. Wild waterfowl are considered the natural reservoir of all influenza A viruses. They have probably carried influenza viruses, with no apparent harm, for centuries. They are known to carry viruses of the H5 and H7 subtypes, but usually in the low pathogenic form. Considerable circumstantial evidence suggests that migratory birds can introduce low pathogenic H5 and H7 viruses to poultry flocks, which then mutate to the highly pathogenic form.

In the past, highly pathogenic viruses have been isolated from migratory birds on very rare occasions involving a few birds, usually found dead within the flight range of a poultry outbreak. This finding long suggested that wild waterfowl are not agents for the onward transmission of these viruses.

Recent events make it likely that some migratory birds are now directly spreading the H5N1 virus in its highly pathogenic form. Further spread to new areas is expected.

6) What is Special About the Current Outbreaks in Poultry?

The current outbreaks of highly pathogenic avian influenza, which began in Southeast Asia in mid-2003, are the largest and most severe on record. Never before in the history of this disease have so many countries been simultaneously affected, resulting in the loss of so many birds.

The causative agent, the H5N1 virus, has proved to be especially tenacious. Despite the death or destruction of an estimated 150 million birds, the virus is now considered endemic in many parts of Indonesia and Vietnam and in some parts of Cambodia, China, Thailand, and possibly also the Lao People's Democratic Republic. Control of the disease in poultry is expected to take several years.

The H5N1 virus is also of particular concern for human health, as explained below.

7) What Symptoms do Birds with Avian Influenza Demonstrate?

Low pathogenicity avian influenza (LPAI) symptoms are typically mild. Decreased food consumption, respiratory signs (coughing and sneezing) and a decrease in egg production might demonstrate the presence of the disease. Birds that are affected with HPAI have a greater level of sickness and may exhibit one or more of the following clinical signs: sudden death; lack of energy and appetite; decreased egg production; soft-shelled or misshapen eggs; swelling; purple discoloration; nasal discharge; coughing, sneezing; lack of coordination and diarrhea.

8) What Should Producers do if their Birds Appear to have Signs of Avian Influenza?

If birds exhibit clinical signs of HPAI or may have been exposed to birds with the disease, producers or bird owners should immediately notify Federal or State animal health officials.

9) Is it Possible for an LPAI Strain to Become Highly Pathogenic?

Some low pathogenic subtypes have the capacity to mutate into more virulent strains. While LPAI is considered lower risk, low pathogenic strains of the virus - the H5 and H7 strains - can mutate to highly pathogenic forms.

10) Is Avian Influenza a Reportable Disease?

HPAI is considered a reportable disease by the World Organization for Animal Health (OIE). OIE has developed animal health standards that classify all H5 and H7 viruses as reportable diseases.

11) Which Countries have been Affected by Outbreaks in Poultry?

From mid-December 2003 through early February 2004, poultry outbreaks caused by the H5N1 virus were reported in eight Asian nations (listed in order of reporting): the Republic of Korea, Vietnam, Japan, Thailand, Cambodia, Lao People's Democratic Republic, Indonesia, and China. Most of these countries had never before experienced an outbreak of highly pathogenic avian influenza in their histories.

In early August 2004, Malaysia reported its first outbreak of H5N1 in poultry, becoming the ninth Asian nation affected. Russia reported its first H5N1 outbreak in poultry in late July 2005, followed by reports of disease in adjacent parts of Kazakhstan in early August. Deaths of wild birds from highly pathogenic H5N1 were reported in both countries. Almost simultaneously, Mongolia reported the detection of H5N1 in dead migratory birds. In October 2005, H5N1 was confirmed in poultry in Turkey and Romania. Outbreaks in wild and domestic birds are under investigation elsewhere.

Japan, the Republic of Korea, and Malaysia have announced control of their poultry outbreaks and are now considered free of the disease.

In the other affected areas, outbreaks are continuing with varying degrees of severity.

12) What are the Implications for Human Health?

The widespread persistence of H5N1 in poultry populations poses two main risks for human health.

The first is the risk of direct infection when the virus passes from poultry to humans, resulting in very severe disease. Of the few avian influenza viruses that have crossed the species barrier to infect humans, H5N1 has caused the largest number of cases of severe disease and death in humans. Unlike normal seasonal influenza, where infection causes only mild respiratory symptoms in most people, the disease caused by H5N1 follows an unusually aggressive clinical course, with rapid deterioration and high fatality. Primary viral pneumonia and multi-organ failure are common. In the present outbreak, more than half of those infected with the virus have died. Most cases have occurred in previously healthy children and young adults.

A second risk, of even greater concern, is that the virus – if given enough opportunities – will change into a form that is highly infectious for humans and spreads easily from person to person. Such a change could mark the start of a global outbreak (a pandemic).

13) What are the Symptoms of Bird Flu in Humans?

Symptoms of bird flu in humans have ranged from typical flu-like symptoms (fever, cough, sore throat and muscle aches) to eye infections, pneumonia, severe respiratory diseases (such as acute respiratory distress), and other severe and life-threatening complications. The symptoms of bird flu may depend on which virus caused the infection.

14) Where have Human Cases Occurred?

In the current outbreak, laboratory-confirmed human cases have been reported in four countries: Cambodia, Indonesia, Thailand, and Vietnam.

Hong Kong has experienced two outbreaks in the past. In 1997, in the first recorded instance of human infection with H5N1, the virus infected 18 people and killed 6 of them. In early 2003, the virus caused two infections, with one death, in a Hong Kong family with a recent travel history to southern China.

15) How do People Become Infected?

Direct contact with infected poultry, or surfaces and objects contaminated by their feces, is presently considered the main route of human infection. To date, most human cases have occurred in rural or periurban areas where many households keep small poultry flocks, which often roam freely, sometimes entering homes or sharing outdoor areas where children play. As infected birds shed large quantities of virus in their feces, opportunities for exposure to infected droppings or to environments contaminated by the virus are abundant under such conditions. Moreover, because many households in Asia depend on poultry for income and food, many families sell or slaughter and consume birds when signs of illness appear in a flock, and this practice has proved difficult to change. Exposure is considered most likely during slaughter, defeathering, butchering, and preparation of poultry for cooking. There is no evidence that properly cooked poultry or eggs can be a source of infection.

16) Does the Virus Spread Easily from Birds to Humans?

No. Though more than 100 human cases have occurred in the current outbreak, this is a small number compared with the huge number of birds affected and the numerous associated opportunities for human exposure, especially in areas where backyard flocks are common. It is not presently understood why some people, and not others, become infected following similar exposures.

17) Does Avian Influenza Threaten Human Health?

LPAI poses no known serious threat to human health, however some strains of HPAI viruses can be infectious to people. Since December 2003, a growing number of Asian countries have reported outbreaks of HPAI in chickens and ducks. Humans also have been affected, most of who had direct contact with infected birds. The rapid spread of HPAI in 2004 and 2005 is historically unprecedented and of growing concern for human health as well as for animal health.

18) What about the Pandemic Risk?

A pandemic can start when three conditions have been met: a new influenza virus subtype emerges; it infects humans, causing serious illness; and it spreads easily and sustainably among humans. The H5N1 virus amply meets the first two conditions: it is a new virus for humans (H5N1 viruses have never circulated widely among people), and it has infected more than 100 humans, killing over half of them. No one will have immunity should an H5N1-like virus emerge.

All prerequisites for the start of a pandemic have therefore been met save one: the establishment of efficient and sustained human-to-human transmission of the virus. The risk that the H5N1 virus will acquire this ability will persist as long as opportunities for human infections occur. These opportunities, in turn, will persist as long as the virus continues to circulate in birds, and this situation could endure for some years to come.

19) What Changes are Needed for H5N1 to Become a Pandemic Vrus?

The virus can improve its transmissibility among humans via two principal mechanisms. The first is a "reassortment" event, in which genetic material is exchanged between human and avian viruses during co-infection of a human or pig. Reassortment could result in a fully transmissible pandemic virus, announced by a sudden surge of cases with explosive spread.

The second mechanism is a more gradual process of adaptive mutation, whereby the capability of the virus to bind to human cells increases during subsequent infections of humans. Adaptive mutation, expressed initially as small clusters of human cases with some evidence of human-to-human transmission, would probably give the world some time to take defensive action.

20) Does HPAI Currently Exist in the United States? Has it Ever Occurred in this Country?

HPAI does not currently exist in the United States. There have been three outbreaks of the disease in poultry in this country--in 1924, 1983 and 2004.

A HPAI epidemic occurred in the northeastern United States in 1983-84. A highly virulent H5 virus produced severe clinical disease and high mortality in chickens, turkeys, and guinea fowl in Pennsylvania and Virginia. Approximately 17 million birds had to be destroyed.

In February 2004, USDA confirmed that an H5N2 strain of avian influenza in a flock of chickens in Texas was consistent with HPAI. There was no evidence of any human health implications of this HPAI virus in Texas. USDA worked with state officials to quickly eradicate the disease. Because of the quick response, the disease was limited to one small flock.

21) What is the H5N1 Bird Flu that has been Reported in Asia and Europe?

Outbreaks of influenza H5N1 occurred among poultry in eight countries in Asia (Cambodia, China, Indonesia, Japan, Laos, South Korea, Thailand, and Vietnam) during late 2003 and early 2004. At that time, more than 100 million birds in the affected countries either died from the disease or were killed in order to try to control the outbreak. By March 2004, the outbreak was reported to be under control. Beginning in late June 2004, however, new outbreaks of influenza H5N1 among poultry were reported by several countries in Asia (Cambodia, China [Tibet], Indonesia, Kazakhastan, Malaysia, Mongolia, Russia [Siberia], Thailand, and Vietnam). It is believed that these outbreaks are ongoing. Most recently, influenza H5N1 has been reported among poultry in Turkey and Romania. Human infections of influenza A (H5N1) have been reported in Cambodia, Indonesia, Thailand, and Vietnam.

22) What is the Significance of Limited Human-to-Human Transmission?

Though rare, instances of limited human-to-human transmission of H5N1 and other avian influenza viruses have occurred in association with outbreaks in poultry and should not be a cause for alarm. In no instance has the virus spread beyond a first generation of close contacts or caused illness in the general community. Data from these incidents suggest that transmission requires very close contact with an ill person. Such incidents must be thoroughly investigated but – provided the investigation indicates that transmission from person to person is very limited – such incidents will not change the WHO overall assessment of the pandemic risk. There have been a number of instances of avian influenza infection occurring among close family members. It is often impossible to determine if human-to-human transmission has occurred since the family members are exposed to the same animal and environmental sources as well as to one another.

23) How Serious is the Current Pandemic Risk?

The risk of pandemic influenza is serious. With the H5N1 virus now firmly entrenched in large parts of Asia, the risk that more human cases will occur will persist. Each additional human case gives the virus an opportunity to improve its transmissibility in humans, and thus develop into a pandemic strain. The recent spread of the virus to poultry and wild birds in new areas further broadens opportunities for human cases to occur. While neither the timing nor the severity of the next pandemic can be predicted, the probability that a pandemic will occur has increased.

24) What is the Risk to Humans from the H5N1 Virus in Asia and Europe?

The H5N1 virus does not usually infect humans. In 1997, however, the first case of spread from a bird to a human was seen during an outbreak of bird flu in poultry in Hong Kong, Special Administrative Region. The virus caused severe respiratory illness in 18 people, 6 of whom died. Since that time, there have been other cases of H5N1 infection among humans. Recent human cases of H5N1 infection that have occurred in Cambodia, Thailand, and Vietnam have coincided with large H5N1 outbreaks in poultry. The World Health Organization (WHO) also has reported human cases in Indonesia. Most of these cases have occurred from contact with infected poultry or contaminated surfaces; however, it is thought that a few cases of human-to-human spread of H5N1 have occurred.

So far, spread of H5N1 virus from person to person has been rare and has not continued beyond one person. However, because all influenza viruses have the ability to change, scientists are concerned that the H5N1 virus one day could be able to infect humans and spread easily from one person to another. Because these viruses do not commonly infect humans, there is little or no immune protection against them in the human population. If the H5N1 virus were able to infect people and spread easily from person to person, an influenza pandemic(worldwide outbreak of disease) could begin. No one can predict when a pandemic might occur. However, experts from around the world are watching the H5N1 situation in Asia very closely and are preparing for the possibility that the virus may begin to spread more easily and widely from person to person.

25) Are There any other Causes for Concern?

Yes. Several.

- Domestic ducks can now excrete large quantities of highly pathogenic virus without showing signs of illness, and are now acting as a "silent" reservoir of the virus, perpetuating transmission to other birds. This adds yet another layer of complexity to control efforts and removes the warning signal for humans to avoid risky behaviours.

- When compared with H5N1 viruses from 1997 and early 2004, H5N1 viruses now circulating are more lethal to experimentally infected mice and to ferrets (a mammalian model) and survive longer in the environment.

- H5N1 appears to have expanded its host range, infecting and killing mammalian species previously considered resistant to infection with avian influenza viruses.

- The behaviour of the virus in its natural reservoir, wild waterfowl, may be changing. The spring 2005 die-off of upwards of 6,000 migratory birds at a nature reserve in central China, caused by highly pathogenic H5N1, was highly unusual and probably unprecedented. In the past, only two large die-offs in migratory birds, caused by highly pathogenic viruses, are known to have occurred: in South Africa in 1961 (H5N3) and in Hong Kong in the winter of 2002–2003 (H5N1).

26) Why are Pandemics Such Dreaded Events?

Influenza pandemics are remarkable events that can rapidly infect virtually all countries. Once international spread begins, pandemics are considered unstoppable, caused as they are by a virus that spreads very rapidly by coughing or sneezing. The fact that infected people can shed virus before symptoms appear adds to the risk of international spread via asymptomatic air travellers.

The severity of disease and the number of deaths caused by a pandemic virus vary greatly, and cannot be known prior to the emergence of the virus. During past pandemics, attack rates reached 25-35% of the total population. Under the best circumstances, assuming that the new virus causes mild disease, the world could still experience an estimated 2 million to 7.4 million deaths (projected from data obtained during the 1957 pandemic). Projections for a more virulent virus are much higher. The 1918 pandemic, which was exceptional, killed at least 40 million people. In the USA, the mortality rate during that pandemic was around 2.5%.

Pandemics can cause large surges in the numbers of people requiring or seeking medical or hospital treatment, temporarily overwhelming health services. High rates of worker absenteeism can also interrupt other essential services, such as law enforcement, transportation, and communications. Because populations will be fully susceptible to an H5N1-like virus, rates of illness could peak fairly rapidly within a given community. This means that local social and economic disruptions may be temporary. They may, however, be amplified in today's closely interrelated and interdependent systems of trade and commerce. Based on past experience, a second wave of global spread should be anticipated within a year.

As all countries are likely to experience emergency conditions during a pandemic, opportunities for inter-country assistance, as seen during natural disasters or localized disease outbreaks, may be curtailed once international spread has begun and governments focus on protecting domestic populations.

27) What are the Most Important Warning Signals that a Pandemic is About to Start?

The most important warning signal comes when clusters of patients with clinical symptoms of influenza, closely related in time and place, are detected, as this suggests human-to-human transmission is taking place. For similar reasons, the detection of cases in health workers caring for H5N1 patients would suggest human-to-human transmission. Detection of such events should be followed by immediate field investigation of every possible case to confirm the diagnosis, identify the source, and determine whether human-to-human transmission is occurring.

Studies of viruses, conducted by specialized WHO reference laboratories, can corroborate field investigations by spotting genetic and other changes in the virus indicative of an improved ability to infect humans. This is why WHO repeatedly asks affected countries to share viruses with the international research community.

28) What is the Status of Vaccine Development and Production?

Vaccines effective against a pandemic virus are not yet available. Vaccines are produced each year for seasonal influenza but will not protect against pandemic influenza. Although a vaccine against the H5N1 virus is under development in several countries, no vaccine is ready for commercial production and no vaccines are expected to be widely available until several months after the start of a pandemic.

Some clinical trials are now under way to test whether experimental vaccines will be fully protective and to determine whether different formulations can economize on the amount of antigen required, thus boosting production capacity. Because the vaccine needs to closely match the pandemic virus, large-scale commercial production will not start until the new virus has emerged and a pandemic has been declared. Current global production capacity falls far short of the demand expected during a pandemic.

29) What Drugs are Available for Treatment?

Two drugs (in the neuraminidase inhibitors class), oseltamivir (commercially known as Tamiflu) and zanamivir (commercially known as Relenza) can reduce the severity and duration of illness caused by seasonal influenza. The efficacy of the neuraminidase inhibitors depends on their administration within 48 hours after symptom onset. For cases of human infection with H5N1, the drugs may improve prospects of survival, if administered early, but clinical data are limited. The H5N1 virus is expected to be susceptible to the neuraminidase inhibitors.

An older class of antiviral drugs, the M2 inhibitors amantadine and rimantadine, could potentially be used against pandemic influenza, but resistance to these drugs can develop rapidly and this could significantly limit their effectiveness against pandemic influenza. Some currently circulating H5N1 strains are fully resistant to these the M2 inhibitors. However, should a new virus emerge through reassortment, the M2 inhibitors might be effective.

For the neuraminidase inhibitors, the main constraints – which are substantial – involve limited production capacity and a price that is prohibitively high for many countries. At present manufacturing capacity, which has recently quadrupled, it will take a decade to produce enough oseltamivir to treat 20% of the world's population. The manufacturing process for oseltamivir is complex and time-consuming, and is not easily transferred to other facilities.

So far, most fatal pneumonia seen in cases of H5N1 infection has resulted from the effects of the virus, and cannot be treated with antibiotics. Nonetheless, since influenza is often complicated by secondary bacterial infection of the lungs, antibiotics could be life-saving in the case of late-onset pneumonia. WHO regards it as prudent for countries to ensure adequate supplies of antibiotics in advance.

30) Can a Pandemic be Prevented?

No one knows with certainty. The best way to prevent a pandemic would be to eliminate the virus from birds, but it has become increasingly doubtful if this can be achieved within the near future.

Following a donation by industry, WHO will have a stockpile of antiviral medications, sufficient for 3 million treatment courses, by early 2006. Recent studies, based on mathematical modelling, suggest that these drugs could be used prophylactically near the start of a pandemic to reduce the risk that a fully transmissible virus will emerge or at least to delay its international spread, thus gaining time to augment vaccine supplies.

The success of this strategy, which has never been tested, depends on several assumptions about the early behaviour of a pandemic virus, which cannot be known in advance. Success also depends on excellent surveillance and logistics capacity in the initially affected areas, combined with an ability to enforce movement restrictions in and out of the affected area. To increase the likelihood that early intervention using the WHO rapid-intervention stockpile of antiviral drugs will be successful, surveillance in affected countries needs to improve, particularly concerning the capacity to detect clusters of cases closely related in time and place.

31) What Strategic Actions are Recommended by WHO?

In August 2005, WHO sent all countries a document outlining recommended strategic actions for responding to the avian influenza pandemic threat. Recommended actions aim to strengthen national preparedness, reduce opportunities for a pandemic virus to emerge, improve the early warning system, delay initial international spread, and accelerate vaccine development.

32) Is the World Adequately Prepared?

No. Despite an advance warning that has lasted almost two years, the world is ill-prepared to defend itself during a pandemic. WHO has urged all countries to develop preparedness plans, but only around 40 have done so. WHO has further urged countries with adequate resources to stockpile antiviral drugs nationally for use at the start of a pandemic. Around 30 countries are purchasing large quantities of these drugs, but the manufacturer has no capacity to fill these orders immediately. On present trends, most developing countries will have no access to vaccines and antiviral drugs throughout the duration of a pandemic.

33) What does CDC Recommend Regarding the H5N1 Bird Flu Outbreak?

In February 2004, CDC provided U.S. health departments with recommendations for enhanced surveillance ("detection") in the U.S. of avian influenza A (H5N1). Follow-up messages, distributed via the Health Alert Network, were sent to the health departments on August 12, 2004, and February 4, 2005; both alerts reminded health departments about how to detect (domestic surveillance), diagnose, and prevent the spread of avian influenza A (H5N1). The alerts also recommended measures for laboratory testing for H5N1 virus. CDC currently advises that travelers to countries with known outbreaks of influenza A (H5N1) avoid poultry farms, contact with animals in live food markets, and any surfaces that appear to be contaminated with feces from poultry or other animals. CDC does not recommend any travel restrictions to affected countries at this time.

34) What is CDC Doing to Prepare for a Possible H5N1 Flu Pandemic?

CDC is taking part in a number of pandemic prevention and preparedness activities, including:

- Providing leadership to the National Pandemic Influenza Preparedness and Response Task Force, created in May 2005 by the Secretary of the U.S. Department of Health and Human Services.

- Working with the Association of Public Health Laboratories on training workshops for state laboratories on the use of special laboratory (molecular) techniques to identify H5 viruses.

- Working with the Council of State and Territorial Epidemiologists and others to help states with their pandemic planning efforts.

- Working with other agencies such as the Department of Defense and the Veterans Administration on antiviral stockpile issues.

- Working with the World Health Organization (WHO) and Vietnamese Ministry of Health to investigate influenza H5N1 in Vietnam and to provide help in laboratory diagnostics and training to local authorities.

- Performing laboratory testing of H5N1 viruses.

- Starting a $5.5 million initiative to improve influenza surveillance in Asia.

- Holding or taking part in training sessions to improve local capacities to conduct surveillance for possible human cases of H5N1 and to detect influenza A H5 viruses by using laboratory techniques.

- Developing and distributing reagents kits to detect the currently circulating influenza A H5N1 viruses.

Working together with WHO and the National Institutes of Health (NIH) on safety testing of vaccine seed candidates and to develop additional vaccine virus seed candidates for influenza A (H5N1) and other subtypes of influenza A virus.

35) What is USDA Doing to Prevent the Introduction of HPAI into the United States?

USDA recognizes that HPAI poses a significant threat to animal health and has the potential to threaten human health. Accordingly, USDA's Animal and Plant Health Inspection Service (APHIS) has safeguards in place to protect against the introduction of HPAI into the United States. APHIS maintains trade restrictions on the importation of poultry and poultry products from countries currently affected by HPAI. These restrictions include:

- Prohibiting the importation of live birds and hatching eggs from H5N1 affected countries.

- Requiring imports of poultry products from East and Southeast Asia be processed or cooked in accordance with a USDA permit prior to importation to lower the risk of HPAI contamination to negligible levels.

- Requiring all imported birds be quarantined at a USDA bird-quarantine facility and be tested for the avian influenza virus before entering the country. This requirement now covers returning U.S.-origin pet birds.

Detection

USDA also works closely with international organizations like the World Organization for Animal Health (OIE), the United Nations' Food and Agriculture Organization (FAO), and World Health Organization (WHO) to assist HPAI-affected countries and other neighboring Asian-Pacific countries with disease prevention, management, and eradication activities. By helping these countries prepare for, manage, or eradicate HPAI (H5N1) outbreaks, USDA can reduce the risk of the disease spreading from overseas to the United States.

APHIS also recognizes that prevention is only one part of a comprehensive strategy and therefore continues to work closely with its Federal, State, and Tribal partners and industry stakeholders to have effective and coordinated emergency response plans at the ready should an outbreak of HPAI occur in the United States.

36) What is USDA Doing to Monitor the U.S. for Avian Influenza Among Birds?

The USDA Animal and Plant Health Inspection Service (APHIS) works with states to monitor and respond to outbreaks of LPAI. APHIS has provided funding and support personnel to states when LPAI has been detected. When HPAI is detected, APHIS personnel are primary responders, due to its infectivity and high mortality rate among poultry. Close attention is also given to two subtypes of LPAI, the H5 and H7 strains, because of the potential for them to mutate into HPAI. The avian influenza strain infecting both birds and humans in Asia is the HPAI H5N1. There is presently no evidence of HPAI H5N1 existing in the U.S. - neither in animals nor humans.

In addition to international import restrictions, APHIS and State veterinarians are specially trained to diagnose foreign animal diseases regularly conduct field investigations of suspicious disease conditions. This surveillance is assisted by university personnel, State animal health officials, USDA-accredited veterinarians, and members of the industry who report suspicious cases. APHIS and State animal health officials work cooperatively with the poultry industry to conduct surveillance at breeding flocks, slaughter plants, live-bird markets, livestock auctions, and poultry dealers.

37) What can Poultry Producers do to Prevent an Avian Influenza Outbreak on their Farms?

Poultry producers should strengthen biosecurity practices to prevent the introduction of avian influenza into their flocks. The following are some sound biosecurity practices:

- Keep an "all-in, all-out" philosophy of flock management. Avoid skimming flocks-birds left behind are exposed to work crews and equipment that may carry poultry disease viruses. Process each lot of birds separately, and clean and disinfect poultry houses between flocks.

- Protect poultry flocks from coming into contact with wild or migratory birds. Keep poultry away from any source of water that may have been contaminated by wild birds.

- Permit only essential workers and vehicles to enter the farm.

- Provide clean clothing and disinfection facilities for employees.

- Thoroughly clean and disinfect equipment and vehicles (including tires and undercarriage) entering and leaving the farm.

- Do not loan to, or borrow equipment or vehicles from, other farms.

- Change footwear and clothing before working with your own flock after visiting another farm or live-bird market or avoid visiting another bird farm if possible.

- Do not bring birds from slaughter channels, especially those from live-bird markets, back to the farm.

If avian influenza is detected, farms must be thoroughly cleaned and disinfected. Avian influenza is inactivated by heat and drying and it is also very sensitive to most disinfectants and detergents. The area to be disinfected must be clear of organic material, which greatly increases the resistance of avian influenza virus' resistance to disinfection.

38) Does Proper Food Handling Prevent Avian Influenza?

The USDA Food Safety and Inspection Service (FSIS) is working to educate the public about safe food handling practices in response to numerous questions from the public about the human risk associated with avian influenza. LPAI, the type commonly found in the U.S., is not transmissible by eating poultry. If HPAI were detected in the U.S., the chance of infected poultry entering the food chain would be extremely low. Nevertheless, proper handling and cooking of poultry provides protection against HPAI, as it does against other viruses and bacteria, including Salmonella and E.coli. USDA continually reminds consumers to practice safe food handling and preparation every day:

- Wash hands before and after handling food;

- Prevent cross-contamination by keeping raw meat, poultry, fish and their juices away from other foods;

- Wash hands, cutting board, knife, and counter tops with hot, soapy water after cutting raw meats;

- Sanitize cutting boards by using a solution of 1 teaspoon chlorine bleach in 1 quart of water and

- Use a food thermometer to ensure food has reached proper temperatures -details available on-line at

www.fsis.usda.gov

Current science indicates that-- as with all foodborne pathogens-- proper cooking of poultry minimizes the risk of illness from consumption of poultry. Using a food thermometer is the only sure way of knowing if your food has reached a high enough temperature to destroy foodborne pathogens including bacteria and viruses. USDA recommends cooking whole birds to 180 °F as measured in the thigh using a food thermometer. When cooking pieces, the breast should reach 170 °F internally. Drumsticks, thighs and wings should be cooked until they reach an internal temperature of 180 °F. Ground turkey and chicken should be cooked to 165° F. The minimum oven temperature to use when cooking poultry is 325 °F. Remember to wash hands with soap and warm water for 20 seconds before and after handling raw poultry.

39) Are Poultry Products from Countries with Avian Influenza Allowed into the United States?

No. Poultry products imported to the U.S. must meet all safety standards applied to foods produced in the U.S. Currently, no poultry from flocks with confirmed cases of high-pathogencity avian influenza or reportable types of low-pathogenicy avian influenza (H5 or H7) are allowed to be exported to the United States.

40) How Does Seasonal Flu Differ from Pandemic Flu?

Seasonal Flu	Pandemic Flu
Outbreaks follow predictable seasonal patterns; occurs annually, usually in winter, in temperate climates	Occurs rarely (three times in 20th century - last in 1968)
Usually some immunity built up from previous exposure	No previous exposure; little or no pre-existing immunity
Healthy adults usually not at risk for serious complications; the very young, the elderly and those with certain underlying health conditions at increased risk for serious complications	Healthy people may be at increased risk for serious complications
Health systems can usually meet public and patient needs	Health systems may be overwhelmed
Vaccine developed based on known flu strains and available for annual flu season	Vaccine probably would not be available in the early stages of a pandemic
Adequate supplies of antivirals are usually available	Effective antivirals may be in limited supply
Average U.S. deaths approximately 36,000/yr	Number of deaths could be quite high (e.g., U.S. 1918 death toll approximately 500,000)
Symptoms: fever, cough, runny nose, muscle pain. Deaths often caused by complications, such as pneumonia.	Symptoms may be more severe and complications more frequent
Generally causes modest impact on society (e.g., some school closing, encouragement of people who are sick to stay home)	May cause major impact on society (e.g. widespread restrictions on travel, closings of schools and businesses, cancellation of large public gatherings)
Manageable impact on domestic and world economy	Potential for severe impact on domestic and world economy

[1] Influenza viruses are grouped into three types, designated A, B, and C. Influenza A and B viruses are of concern for human health. Only influenza A viruses can cause pandemics.

[2] The H subtypes are epidemiologically most important, as they

govern the ability of the virus to bind to and enter cells, where multiplication of the virus then occurs. The N subtypes govern the release of newly formed virus from the cells.

Note: The source material for this chapter was obtained from the World Health Organization, the Centers for Disease Control and Prevention, and the United States Department of Agriculture websites.

CHAPTER SEVEN

AVIAN INFLUENZA INFECTION IN HUMANS

Although avian influenza A viruses usually do not infect humans, several instances of human infections have been reported since 1997. Most cases of avian influenza infection in humans are thought to have resulted from direct contact with infected poultry or contaminated surfaces. However, there is still a lot to learn about how different subtypes and strains of avian influenza virus might affect humans. For example, it is not known how the distinction between low pathogenic and highly pathogenic strains might impact the health risk to humans. (For more information, see "Low Pathogenic versus Highly Pathogenic Avian Influenza Viruses" on the CDC Influenza Viruses Web page.

Because of concerns about the potential for more widespread infection in the human population, public health authorities closely monitor outbreaks of human illness associated with avian influenza. To date, human infections with avian influenza A viruses detected since 1997 have not resulted in sustained human-to-human transmission. However, because influenza A viruses have the potential to change and gain the ability to spread easily between people, monitoring for human infection and person-to-person transmission is important.

Instances of Avian Influenza Infections in Humans

Confirmed instances of avian influenza viruses infecting humans since 1997 include:

- H5N1, Hong Kong, Special Administrative Region, 1997: Highly pathogenic avian influenza A (H5N1) infections occurred in both poultry and humans. This was the first time an avian influenza A virus transmission directly from birds to humans had been found. During this outbreak, 18 people were hospitalized and six of them died. To control the outbreak, authorities killed about 1.5 million chickens to remove the source of the virus. Scientists determined that the virus spread primarily from birds to humans, though rare person-to-person infection was noted.

- H9N2, China and Hong Kong, Special Administrative Region, 1999: Low pathogenic avian influenza A (H9N2) virus infection was confirmed in two children and resulted in uncomplicated influenza-like illness. Both patients recovered, and no additional cases were confirmed. The source is unknown, but the evidence suggested that poultry was the source of infection and the main mode of transmission was from bird to human. However, the possibility of person-to-person transmission could not be ruled out. Several additional human H9N2 infections were reported from China in 1998-99.

- H7N2, Virginia , 2002: Following an outbreak of H7N2 among poultry in the Shenandoah Valley poultry production area, one person was found to have serologic evidence of infection with H7N2.

- H5N1, China and Hong Kong, Special Administrative Region, 2003: Two cases of highly pathogenic avian influenza A (H5N1) infection occurred among members of a Hong Kong family that had traveled to China . One person recovered, the other died. How or where these two family members were infected was not determined. Another family member died of a respiratory illness in China , but no testing was done.

- H7N7, Netherlands, 2003: The Netherlands reported outbreaks of influenza A (H7N7) in poultry on several farms. Later, infections were reported among pigs and humans. In total, 89 people were confirmed to have H7N7 influenza virus infection associated with this poultry outbreak. These cases occurred mostly among poultry workers. H7N7-associated illness included 78 cases of conjunctivitis (eye infections) only; 5 cases of conjunctivitis and influenza-like illnesses with cough, fever, and muscle aches; 2 cases of influenza-like illness only; and 4 cases that were classified as "other." There was one death among the 89 total cases. It occurred in a veterinarian who visited one of the affected farms and developed acute respiratory distress syndrome and complications related to H7N7 infection. The majority of these cases occurred as a result of direct contact with infected poultry; however, Dutch authorities reported three possible instances of transmission from poultry workers to family members. Since then, no other instances of H7N7 infection among humans have been reported.

- H9N2, Hong Kong, Special Administrative Region, 2003: Low pathogenic avian influenza A (H9N2) infection was confirmed in a child in Hong Kong . The child was hospitalized and recovered.

- H7N2, New York, 2003: In November 2003, a patient with serious underlying medical conditions was admitted to a hospital in New York with respiratory symptoms. One of the initial laboratory tests identified an influenza A virus that was thought to be H1N1. The patient recovered and went home after a few weeks. Subsequent confirmatory tests conducted in March 2004 showed that the patient had been infected with avian influenza A (H7N2) virus.

- H7N3 in Canada, 2004: In February 2004, human infections of highly pathogenic avian influenza A (H7N3) among poultry workers were associated with an H7N3 outbreak among poultry. The H7N3-associated, mild illnesses consisted of eye infections.

- H5N1, Thailand and Vietnam, 2004, and other outbreaks in Asia during 2004 and 2005: In January 2004, outbreaks of highly pathogenic influenza A (H5N1) in Asia were first reported by the World Health Organization. Visit the Avian Influenza section of the World Health Organization Web site for more information and updates.

Symptoms of Avian Influenza in Humans

The reported symptoms of avian influenza in humans have ranged from typical influenza-like symptoms (e.g., fever, cough, sore throat, and muscle aches) to eye infections (conjunctivitis), pneumonia, acute respiratory distress, viral pneumonia, and other severe and life-threatening complications.

Antiviral Agents for Influenza

Four different influenza antiviral drugs (amantadine, rimantadine, oseltamivir, and zanamivir) are approved by the U.S. Food and Drug Administration (FDA) for the treatment of influenza; three are approved for prophylaxis. All four have activity against influenza A viruses. However, sometimes influenza strains can become resistant to these drugs, and therefore the drugs may not always be effective. For example, analyses of some of the 2004 H5N1 viruses isolated from poultry and humans in Asia have shown that the viruses are resistant to two of the medications (amantadine and rimantadine). Monitoring of avian influenza A viruses for resistance to influenza antiviral medications is ongoing.

Note: The source material for this chapter was obtained from the Centers for Disease Control and Prevention website.

CHAPTER EIGHT

TRANSMISSION OF INFLUENZA A VIRUSES BETWEEN ANIMALS AND PEOPLE

Influenza A viruses have infected many different animals, including ducks, chickens, pigs, whales, horses, and seals. However, certain subtypes of influenza A virus are specific to certain species, except for birds, which are hosts to all known subtypes of influenza A. Subtypes that have caused widespread illness in people either in the past or currently are H3N2, H2N2, H1N1, and H1N2. H1N1 and H3N2 subtypes also have caused outbreaks in pigs, and H7N7 and H3N8 viruses have caused outbreaks in horses.

Influenza A viruses normally seen in one species sometimes can cross over and cause illness in another species. For example, until 1998, only H1N1 viruses circulated widely in the U.S. pig population. However, in 1998, H3N2 viruses from humans were introduced into the pig population and caused widespread disease among pigs. Most recently, H3N8 viruses from horses have crossed over and caused outbreaks in dogs.

Avian influenza A viruses may be transmitted from animals to humans in two main ways:

- Directly from birds or from avian virus-contaminated environments to people.

- Through an intermediate host, such as a pig.

Influenza A viruses have eight separate gene segments. The segmented genome allows influenza A viruses from different species to mix and create a new influenza A virus if viruses from two different species infect the same person or animal. For example, if a pig were infected with a human influenza A virus and an avian influenza A virus at the same time, the new replicating viruses could mix existing genetic information (reassortment) and produce a new virus that had most of the genes from the human virus, but a hemagglutinin and/or neuraminidase from the avian virus. The resulting new virus might then be able to infect humans and spread from person to person, but it would have surface proteins (hemagglutinin and/or neuraminidase) not previously seen in influenza viruses that infect humans.

This type of major change in the influenza A viruses is known as antigenic shift. Antigenic shift results when a new influenza A subtype to which most people have little or no immune protection infects humans. If this new virus causes illness in people and can be transmitted easily from person to person, an influenza pandemic can occur.

It is possible that the process of genetic reassortment could occur in a human who is co-infected with avian influenza A virus and a human strain of influenza A virus. The genetic information in these viruses could reassort to create a new virus with a hemagglutinin from the avian virus and other genes from the human virus. Theoretically, influenza A viruses with a hemagglutinin against which humans have little or no immunity that have reassorted with a human influenza virus are more likely to result in sustained human-to-human transmission and pandemic influenza. Therefore, careful evaluation of influenza viruses recovered from humans who are infected with avian influenza is very important to identify reassortment if it occurs.

Although it is unusual for people to get influenza virus infections directly from animals, sporadic human infections and outbreaks caused by certain avian influenza A viruses and pig influenza viruses have been reported. These sporadic human infections and outbreaks, however, rarely result in sustained transmission among humans.

Note: The source material for this chapter was obtained from the Centers for Disease Control and Prevention website.

CHAPTER NINE

SPREAD OF AVIAN INFLUENZA VIRUSES AMONG BIRDS

Avian influenza viruses circulate among birds worldwide. Certain birds, particularly water birds, act as hosts for influenza viruses by carrying the virus in their intestines and shedding it. Infected birds shed virus in saliva, nasal secretions, and feces. Susceptible birds can become infected with avian influenza virus when they have contact with contaminated nasal, respiratory, or fecal material from infected birds. Fecal-to-oral transmission is the most common mode of spread between birds.

Most often, the wild birds that are host to the virus do not get sick, but they can spread influenza to other birds. Infection with certain avian influenza A viruses (for example, some H5 and H7 strains) can cause widespread disease and death among some species of domesticated birds.

Avian Influenza Outbreaks in Poultry

Domesticated birds may become infected with avian influenza virus through direct contact with infected waterfowl or other infected poultry, or through contact with surfaces (such as dirt or cages) or materials (such as water or feed) that have been contaminated with virus. People, vehicles, and other inanimate objects such as cages can be vectors for the spread of influenza virus from one farm to another. When this happens, avian influenza outbreaks can occur among poultry.

Avian influenza outbreaks among poultry occur worldwide from time to time. Since 1997, for example, more than 16 outbreaks of H5 and H7 influenza have occurred among poultry in the United States. The U.S. Department of Agriculture monitors these outbreaks.

Low pathogenic forms of avian influenza viruses are responsible for most avian influenza outbreaks in poultry. Such outbreaks usually result in either no illness or mild illness (e.g., chickens producing fewer or no eggs), or low levels of mortality.

When highly pathogenic influenza H5 or H7 viruses cause outbreaks, between 90% and 100% of poultry can die from infection. Animal health officials carefully monitor avian influenza outbreaks in domestic birds for several reasons:

- the potential for low pathogenic H5 and H7 viruses to evolve into highly pathogenic forms

- the potential for rapid spread and significant illness and death among poultry during outbreaks of highly pathogenic avian influenza

- the economic impact and trade restrictions from a highly pathogenic avian influenza outbreak

- the possibility that avian influenza could be transmitted to humans

When avian influenza outbreaks occur in poultry, quarantine and depopulation (or culling) and surveillance around affected flocks is the preferred control and eradication option.

For More Information about Avian Influenza Viruses, Visit:

- The United States Department of Agriculture Animal and Plant Health Inspection Service (APHIS) bird biosecurity Web site

- The Avian Influenza page of the World Health Organization Animal Health and Production Division (FAQ) Web site

- The Avian Influenza page of the World Health Organization for Animal Health (OIE) Web site

Note: The source material for this chapter was obtained from the Centers of Disease Control and Prevention website.

CHAPTER TEN

INFLUENZA (FLU) ANTIVIRAL DRUGS AND RELATED INFORMATION

What Drugs are Available?

Four drugs are available to treat and/or prevent influenza. They are amantadine and rimantadine, zanamivir, and oseltamivir.

How Do They Work?

In 1976, the Food and Drug Administration (FDA) approved amantadine to both treat and prevent influenza type A in adults and children 1 year old or older. FDA approved rimantadine-a derivative of amantadine-in 1993 to treat and prevent influenza infection in adults and prevent influenza in children.

These two drugs act against influenza A viruses but not against influenza B viruses. These compounds inhibit the activity of the influenza virus M2 protein, which forms a channel in the virus membrane. As a result, the virus cannot replicate (make copies of itself) after it enters a cell. The drug manufacturers recommend daily doses for using amantadine and rimantadine to treat and prevent the flu in different age groups. Researchers, however, have not adequately evaluated amantadine and rimantadine in children younger than 1 year old.

In 1999, FDA approved two additional drugs to fight the flu: Relenza (zanamivir) and Tamiflu (oseltamivir), the first of a new class of antiviral drugs called neuraminidase inhibitors.

The surfaces of influenza viruses are dotted with neuraminidase proteins. Neuraminidase, an enzyme, breaks the bonds that hold new virus particles to the outside of an infected cell. Once the enzyme breaks these bonds, this sets free new viruses that can infect other cells and spread infection. Neuraminidase inhibitors block the enzyme's activity and prevent new virus particles from being released, thereby limiting the spread of infection.

Are These Drugs Effective Against Any Kind of Influenza Virus?

Rimantadine and amantadine are effective only against type A influenza. Zanamivir and oseltamivir inhibit both influenza A and B viruses.

Who Should Consider Using these Drugs?

Amantadine is approved for treating and preventing uncomplicated influenza A virus infection in adults and children who are 1 year of age or older. Rimantadine is approved for treating and preventing uncomplicated influenza virus A infection in adults and for preventing, but not treating, such infections in children.

Zanamivir is approved only for treating uncomplicated influenza virus infection in people 7 years of age and older who have not had symptoms for more than 2 days.

Oseltamivir is approved for treating uncomplicated influenza virus infection in people 1 year of age or older who have not had symptoms for more than 2 days. A pediatric liquid formulation is available for oseltamivir. Oseltamivir also is approved for preventing influenza A and B in people 13 years and older. Currently, oseltamivir is the only neuraminidase inhibitor approved to prevent the flu.

How are these Drugs Administered?

Amantadine and rimantadine are taken orally in pill form.

Zanamivir, available as a dry powder, can be inhaled using a device known as a "Diskhaler." The recommended dosage is two inhalations twice a day, morning and night, for 5 days.

Oseltamivir is available as a pill and for adults is taken twice daily for 5 days. For children, the dose of oseltamivir depends on the child's weight. A liquid suspension of oseltamivir can be taken by children or adults who cannot swallow a capsule.

How Much Do These Drugs Help?

Studies have shown that all four drugs can reduce the duration of flu symptoms by 1 day if taken within 2 days of the onset of the illness. There is no information about how effective these drugs are if treatment is started more than 2 days after onset of flu symptoms.

When taken as directed to prevent the flu, oseltamivir can significantly reduce your chance of getting the disease if there is a flu outbreak in your family or community.

Amantadine and rimantadine have been reported to prevent the spread of influenza A outbreaks primarily in nursing homes. If someone in your family is diagnosed with influenza, taking one of these drugs may reduce your chances of getting the disease.

What Other Benefits Might They Have?

None of the four drugs has been shown to effectively prevent serious influenza-related complications such as bacterial or viral pneumonia. Studies of the use of zanamivir in families and in nursing homes at risk for influenza infection, however, resulted in the reduced use of antibiotics, which are frequently prescribed to treat these serious complications.

What About Side Effects?

The neuraminidase inhibitors generally cause fewer side effects than the older flu drugs. The most common side effects seen with oseltamivir are nausea and vomiting. In some people, zanamivir can cause wheezing or serious breathing problems that need prompt treatment. The other most common side effects seen with zanamivir include headache and diarrhea. Amantadine and rimantadine can cause side effects such as insomnia and anxiety, nausea or loss of appetite. In some cases, severe side effects such as seizures have been reported.

Your health care provider or pharmacist can discuss with you a more complete list of possible side effects.

Should Certain People Not Take These Drugs?

People allergic to these drugs or their ingredients should not take them.

Zanamivir generally is not recommended for people with chronic respiratory diseases such as asthma or chronic obstructive pulmonary disease (COPD). In clinical studies, some patients with mild or moderate asthma or COPD had bronchospasm (wheezing) after taking zanamivir. If you have an underlying respiratory disease and have been prescribed zanamivir, your health care provider should instruct you to have a fast-acting inhaled bronchodilator available for use when taking the drug.

The dosage of oseltamivir may need to be adjusted if you have any type of kidney disease.

None of these drugs is recommended for routine use during pregnancy or nursing. These drugs have not been evaluated in pregnant women, and researchers do not know the effects these drugs could have on the unborn child.

In laboratory and in limited clinical studies, there have been no reported interactions of the neuraminidase inhibitors with other drugs.

For complete safety information about these drugs, talk with your pharmacist or health care provider.

Can Influenza Viruses Develop Resistance To These Drugs?

When either amantadine or rimantadine is used for therapy, drug-resistant flu viruses may appear in about one-third of patients.

Laboratory studies have shown that influenza A and B viruses can develop resistance to zanamivir and oseltamivir. Surveillance for neuraminidase inhibitor-resistance has been started.

How Do the Flu Drugs Compare?

No study to date has directly compared the effectiveness of zanamivir, oseltamivir, amantadine, and rimantadine for treating influenza A or zanamivir and oseltamivir for treating influenza A or B. The available information suggests that these four drugs are similarly effective in reducing the duration of uncomplicated acute illness due to influenza A.

Zanamivir and oseltamivir differ from amantadine and rimantadine in terms of their side effects and cost. Use of amantadine, and to a lesser extent rimantadine, has been associated with central nervous system side effects including nervousness, anxiety, insomnia, and lightheadedness. These side effects have not been associated with zanamivir or oseltamivir. On the other hand, zanamivir and oseltamivir are significantly more expensive than either rimantadine or amantadine. All four drugs are available by prescription only, and it is best to consult with your health care provider to determine what drug might be best for you.

Contacts for More Information:

Information on availability of influenza vaccine:
Food and Drug Administration
Center for Biologics Evaluation and Research
Office of Communication, Training & Manufacturers Assistance
301-827-1800. Fax: 301-827-3843
octma@cber.fda.gov

Information on drugs used to treat influenza:
Food and Drug Administration
Center for Drug Evaluation and Research
Drug Information Line
888-info-FDA or 301-827-4573. Fax: 301-827-4577
druginfo@cder.fda.gov

Information on influenza prevention and control:
Centers for Disease Control and Prevention
Public Inquiries Office
800-311-3435 or 404-639-3311. Fax: 770-488-4995
inquiry@cdc.gov

Influenza Information From Other Web Sites

- FDA Flu Information Page. Information on flu prevention and treatment with vaccines and antiviral drugs.
  http://www.fda.gov/oc/opacom/hottopics/flu.html

- Influenza (flu): Protect yourselves and your loved ones. Information for consumers and healthcare professionals from the Centers for Disease Control and Prevention (CDC).
  http://www.cdc.gov/flu/

- World Health Organization (WHO) Influenza Information. This web page provides links to WHO fact sheets, plus global surveillance and outbreak information.
  http://www.who.int/csr/disease/influenza/en/

- National Institute of Allergy and Infectious Diseases. NIAID's flu and cold publications page.
  http://www.niaid.nih.gov/publications/flu.htm

- National Vaccine Program Office Influenza pandemics can occur when a novel strain of virus causes an epidemic that spreads over a wide geographic area and affects an exceptionally high proportion of the population. This web site contains information about influenza, pandemics, and the Draft Pandemic Influenza Preparedness and Response Plan.
  http://www.hhs.gov/nvpo/pandemics/index.html

Note: The source material for this chapter was obtained from the National Institute of Allergy and Infectious Diseases website.

CHAPTER ELEVEN

TRAVELING IN A WORLD WITH AVIAN INFLUENZA

According to the World Health Organization (WHO), the Ministry of Health in Thailand has reported its second laboratory-confirmed human case of avian influenza A (H5N1) since October 2004. The infection has been linked to direct contact with diseased poultry during slaughter.

The Ministry of Health in Indonesia has reported two additional laboratory-confirmed human cases of avian influenza A (H5N1). Both infections have been linked to exposure to diseased poultry.

Since January 2004, human cases of avian influenza A (H5N1) have been reported from Vietnam, Thailand, Cambodia, and Indonesia, with some cases resulting in death. Most human avian influenza cases have been reported among patients who had direct contact with poultry or who live in areas where poultry are present.

During 2005, outbreaks of H5N1 infection among poultry and other birds have been confirmed in Cambodia, China, Croatia, Indonesia, Kazakhstan, Romania, Russia, Thailand, Turkey, and Vietnam. Mongolia has reported outbreaks of H5N1 in wild, migratory birds. Poultry outbreaks were also reported in Malaysia and Laos during 2004. Most cases of H5N1 infection in humans are thought to have occurred from direct contact with infected poultry in the affected countries. Therefore, when possible, care should be taken to avoid contact with live, well-appearing, sick, or dead poultry and with any surfaces that may have been contaminated by poultry or their feces or secretions. Transmission of H5N1 viruses to two persons through consumption of uncooked duck blood may also have occurred in

Vietnam in 2005. Uncooked poultry or poultry products, including blood, should not be consumed.

CDC remains in communication with WHO and continues to closely monitor the H5N1 situation in countries reporting human cases and poultry outbreaks.

The threat of novel influenza subtypes such as influenza A (H5N1) will be greatly increased if the virus gains the ability to spread from one human to another. Such transmission has not yet been observed. However, a few cases of limited person-to-person spread of H5N1 viruses have been reported, with no instances of transmission continuing beyond one person. For example, one instance of probable person-to-person transmission associated with close contact between an ill child and her mother is thought to have occurred in Thailand in September 2004.

H5N1 infections in humans can cause serious disease and death. An inactivated vaccine to protect humans against influenza A (H5N1) is not yet available, but a candidate vaccine is undergoing human clinical trials in the United States. The H5N1 viruses currently infecting birds and some humans in Asia are resistant to amantadine and rimantadine, two antiviral medications commonly used to treat influenza. The H5N1 viruses are susceptible to the antiviral medications oseltamivir and zanamivir, but the effectiveness of these drugs when used for treatment of H5N1 virus infection is unknown.

CDC has not recommended that the general public avoid travel to any of the countries affected by H5N1. Persons visiting areas with reports of outbreaks of H5N1 among poultry or of human H5N1 cases can reduce their risk of infection by observing the following measures:

Before Any International Travel to an Area Affected by H5N1 Avian Influenza:

- Visit CDC's Travelers' Health website on Southeast Asia at http://www.cdc.gov/travel/seasia.htm to educate yourself and others who may be traveling with you about any disease risks and CDC health recommendations for international travel in areas you plan to visit. For other information about avian influenza, see this website:

  http://www.cdc.gov/flu/avian/index.htm.

- Be sure you are up to date with all your vaccinations, and see your doctor or health-care provider, ideally 4-6 weeks before travel, to get any additional vaccination medications or information you may need.

- Assemble a travel health kit containing basic first aid and medical supplies. Be sure to include a thermometer and alcohol-based hand gel for hand hygiene.

- Identify in-country health-care resources in advance of your trip.

- Check your health insurance plan or get additional insurance that covers medical evacuation in case you become sick. Information about medical evacuation services is provided on the U.S. Department of State web page Medical Information for Americans Traveling Abroad, at http://travel.state.gov/travel/tips/health/health_1185.html.

During Travel to an Affected Area:

- Avoid all direct contact with poultry, including touching well-appearing, sick, or dead chickens and ducks. Avoid places such as poultry farms and bird markets where live poultry are raised or kept, and avoid handling surfaces contaminated with poultry feces or secretions.

- As with other infectious illnesses, one of the most important preventive practices is careful and frequent handwashing. Cleaning your hands often with soap and water removes potentially infectious material from your skin and helps prevent disease transmission. Waterless alcohol-based hand gels may be used when soap is not available and hands are not visibly soiled.

- Influenza viruses are destroyed by heat; therefore, as a precaution, all foods from poultry, including eggs and poultry blood, should be thoroughly cooked.

- If you become sick with symptoms such as a fever, difficulty breathing, or cough, or with any illness that requires prompt medical attention, a U.S. consular officer can assist you in locating medical services and informing your family or friends. Inform your health care provider of any possible exposures to avian influenza. You should defer further travel until you are free of symptoms, unless your travel is health-related.

After Your Return:

- Monitor your health for 10 days.

- If you become ill with fever and develop a cough, sore throat, or difficulty breathing or if you develop any illness with fever during this 10-day period, consult a health-care provider.

Before you visit a health-care setting, tell the provider the following: 1) your symptoms, 2) where you traveled, and 3) if you have had direct contact with poultry. This way, he or she can be aware that you have traveled to an area reporting avian influenza.

- Do not travel while ill, unless you are seeking medical care. Limiting contact with others as much as possible can help prevent the spread of an infectious illness.

For more information about H5N1 infections in humans, visit the World Health Organization avian influenza website at http://www.who.int/csr/disease/avian_influenza/en/ and the CDC Avian Influenza site, http://www.cdc.gov/flu/avian/index.htm.

For information about CDC recommendations for enhanced surveillance, diagnostic evaluation, and infection control precautions for H5N1, see

http://www.cdc.gov/flu/avian/professional/han020405.htm.

For more information about CDC's health recommendations for travel to Asia, see

http://www.cdc.gov/travel/seasia.htm and http://www.cdc.gov/travel/eastasia.htm.

Note: The source material for this chapter was obtained from the Centers for Disease Control and Prevention website.

CHAPTER TWELVE

TRANSCRIPT OF PRESIDENT BUSH'S SPEECH ON PANDEMIC FLU STRATEGY

On Tuesday, November 1, 2005, President Bush gave a speech at the National Institutes of Health stating that the United States must be prepared to identify to Bird Flu outbreaks anywhere in the world, and must be in a position to respond in the event that a pandemic occurs in the United States. The fact that the President gave a speech on this subject highlights the importance of the issue.

Following is a transcript of his speech.

"Thank you all.

Michael, thank you very much for your introduction. And thanks for the warm reception here at the National Institutes of Health. It's good to be back here again.

For more than a century, the NIH has been at the forefront of this country's efforts to prevent, detect and treat disease. And I appreciate the good work you're doing here.

This is an important facility, it's an important complex. The people who work here are really important to the security of this nation.

The scientists who have been supported by the folks who work here have developed and improved vaccines for meningitis and whooping cough and measles and mumps and rubella and chicken pox and other infectious diseases. Because of the revolutionary advances in medicine pioneered with the help of the NIH, Americans no longer fear these dreaded diseases. Many lives have been saved.

At this moment, the men and women of NIH are working to protect the American people from another danger: the risk of avian and pandemic influenza.

Today I've come to talk about our nation's efforts to address this vital issue to the health and the safety of all Americans. I'm here to discuss our strategy to prevent and protect the American people from possible outbreak.

I appreciate the members of my Cabinet who are here -- more importantly, I appreciate the hard work you've done on this issue -- Secretary Rice, Secretary Johanns, Secretary Mineta, Secretary Nicholson, Secretary Chertoff.

I appreciate the fact that Dr. J.W. Lee, director general of the World Health Organization, has joined us.

Dr. Lee, thank you for being here.

I want to recognize Dr. David Nabarro, the senior United Nations system coordinator for avian and human influenza.

Thanks for being here.

You're about to hear me talk about the international scope of response and protection necessary to protect not only our own people but people around the world. And the fact that these two gentlemen are here is an important signal.

I want to thank Dr. Elias Zerhouni, who's the director of NIH.

Doing a fine job.

I want to thank Julie Gerberding, who's the director of the Centers for Disease Control and Prevention.

appreciate Dr. Rich Carmona, the U.S. surgeon general; Dr. Tony Fauci, director of the National Institute of Allergy and Infectious Diseases.

I want to thank Dr. Bruce Gellen, director of the National Vaccine Program Office.

I want to thank Dr. Andy Von Eschenbach, who's the acting director of the FDA and the director of the National Cancer Institute.

I appreciate all the members of the health care community who have joined us today.

I want to thank state and local officials who are here.

I particularly want to thank Senators Specter and Kennedy for coming, as well as Congressmen Linder, Burgess and Price. I appreciate you all taking time to be here.

Most Americans are familiar with the influenza or the flu, a respiratory illness that makes hundreds of thousands of people sick every year. This fall as the flu season approaches, millions of our fellow citizens are once again visiting their doctors for the annual flu shot. I had mine.

For most, this is simply a precautionary measure to avoid the fever or sore throat or muscle aches that come with the flu. Seasonal flu is extremely dangerous for some: people whose immune systems have been weakened by age or illness. But it is not usually life- threatening for most healthy people.

Pandemic flu is another matter. Pandemic flu occurs when a new strain of influenza emerges that can be transmitted easily from person to person and for which there's little or no natural immunity.

Unlike seasonal flu, most people have not built up resistance to it. And unlike seasonal flu, it can kill those who are young and health as well as those who are frail and sick.

At this moment there is no pandemic influenza in the United States or the world, but if history is our guide there's reason to be concerned. In the last century, our country and the world have been hit by three influenza pandemics, and viruses from birds contributed to all of them.

The first, which struck in 1918, killed over half a million Americans and more than 20 million people across the globe. One-third of the U.S. population was infected, and life expectancy in our country was reduced by 13 years.

The 1918 pandemic was followed by pandemics in 1957 and 1968 which killed tens of thousands of Americans and millions across the world.

Three years ago, the world had a preview of the disruption an influenza pandemic can cause when a previously unknown virus called SARS appeared in rural China. When an infected doctor carried the virus out of China, it spread to Vietnam and Singapore and Canada within a month. Before long, the SARS virus had spread to nearly 30 countries on six continents. It infected more than 8,000 people and killed nearly 800.

One elderly woman brought the virus from Hong Kong to Toronto, where it quickly spread to her son and then to others. Eventually, four others arrived with the virus and hundreds of Canadians fell ill with SARS and dozens died.

By one estimate the SARS outbreak cost the Asian Pacific region about $40 billion.

The airline industry was hit particularly hard, with air travel to Asia dropping 45 percent in the year after the outbreak.

All this was caused by a limited outbreak of a virus that infected thousands and lasted about six months. A global influenza pandemic that infects millions and lasts from one to three years could be far worse.

Scientists and doctors cannot tell us where or when the next pandemic will strike or how severe it'll be, but most agree: At some point, we are likely to face another pandemic.

And the scientific community is increasingly concerned by a new influenza virus known as H5N1, or avian flu, that is now spreading through bird populations across Asia and has recently reached Europe.

This new strain of influenza has infected domesticated birds like ducks and chickens as well as long-range migratory birds.

In 1997, the first recorded outbreak among people took place in Hong Kong when 18 people became infected and six died from the disease. Public health officials in the region took aggressive action and successively contained the spread of the virus.

Avian flu struck again in late 2003 and has infected over 120 people, in Thailand, Cambodia, Vietnam and Indonesia and killed more than 60.

That's a fatality rate of about 50 percent.

At this point we do not have evidence that a pandemic is imminent. Most of the people in Southeast Asia who got sick were handling infected birds. And while the avian flu virus has spread from Asia to Europe, there are no reports of infected birds, animals or people in the United States.

Even if the virus does eventually appear on our shores in birds, that does not mean people in our country will be infected. Avian flu is still primarily an animal disease. And as of now, unless people come into direct sustained contact with infected birds, it is unlikely they will come down with avian flu.

While avian flu has not yet acquired the ability to spread easily from human to human there is still cause for vigilance. The virus has developed some characteristics needed to cause a pandemic: It has demonstrated the ability to infect human beings and it has produced a fatal illness in humans.

If the virus were to develop the capacity for sustained human-to-human transmission, it could spread quickly across the globe.

Our country has been given fair warning of this danger to our homeland and time to prepare.

It's my responsibility as the president to take measures now to protect the American people from the possible that human-to-human transmission may occur. So several months ago I directed all relevant departments and agencies in the federal government to take steps to address the threat of avian and pandemic flu.

Since that time, my administration has developed a comprehensive national strategy, with concrete measures we can take to prepare for influenza pandemic. Today, I'm announcing key elements of that strategy.

Our strategy is designed to meet three critical goals: first, we must detect outbreaks that occur anywhere in the world; second, we must protect the American people by stockpiling vaccines and antiviral drugs, and improve our ability to rapidly produce new vaccines against a pandemic strain; and third, we must be ready to respond at the federal, state and local levels in the event that a pandemic reaches our shores.

To meet these three goals, our strategy will require the combined efforts of government officials in public health and medical, veterinary and law enforcement communities and the private sector.

It will require the active participation of the American people.

And it will require the immediate attention of the United States Congress so we can have the resources in place to begin implementing this strategy right away.

The first part of our strategy is to detect outbreaks before they spread across the world. In the fight against avian and pandemic flu, early detection is our first line of defense.

A pandemic is a lot like a forest fire: If caught early it might be extinguished with limited damage; if allowed to smolder undetected it can grow to an inferno that spreads quickly beyond our ability to control it.

So we're taking immediate steps to ensure early warning of an avian or pandemic flu outbreak among animals or humans anywhere in the world.

In September at the United Nations, I announced a new international partnership on avian and pandemic influenza, a global network of surveillance and preparedness that will help us to detect and respond quickly to any outbreaks of the disease.

The partnership requires participating countries that face an outbreak to immediately share information and provide samples to the World Health Organization.

By requiring transparency, we can respond more rapidly to dangerous outbreaks.

Since we announced this global initiative, the response from across the world has been very positive. Already 88 countries and nine international organizations have joined the effort.

Senior officials from participating governments recently convened the partnership's first meeting here in Washington.

Together, we're working to control and monitor avian flu in Asia and to ensure that all nations have structures in place to recognize and report outbreaks before they spread beyond human control.

I've requested $251 million from Congress to help our foreign partners train local medical personnel, expand their surveillance and testing capacity, draw up preparedness plans, and take other vital actions to detect and contain outbreaks.

A flu pandemic would have global consequences, so no nation can afford to ignore this threat, and every nation has responsibilities to detect and stop its spread.

Here in the United States we're doing our part. To strengthen domestic surveillance, my administration is launching the National

Biosurveillance Initiative. This initiative will help us rapidly detect, quantify and respond to outbreaks of disease in humans and animals, and deliver information quickly to state and local and national and international public health officials.

By creating systems that provide continuous situational awareness, we're more likely to be able to stop, slow or limit the spread of a pandemic and save American lives.

The second part of our strategy is to protect the American people by stockpiling vaccines and antiviral drugs and accelerating development of new vaccine technologies.

One of the challenges presented by a pandemic is that scientists need a sample of the new strain before they can produce a vaccine against it. This means it is difficult to produce a pandemic vaccine before the pandemic actually appears. And so there may not be a vaccine capable of fully immunizing our citizens from the new influenza virus during the first several months of a pandemic.

To help protect our citizens during these early months, when a fully effective vaccine would not be available, we're taking a number of immediate steps.

Researchers here at the NIH have developed a vaccine based on the current strain of the avian flu virus. The vaccine is already in clinical trials.

And I'm asking that the Congress fund $1.2 billion for the Department of Health and Human Services to purchase enough doses of this vaccine for manufacturers to vaccinate 20 million people.

This vaccine would not be a perfect match to the pandemic flu because the pandemic strain would probably differ somewhat from the avian flu virus it grew from. But a vaccine against the current avian flu virus would likely offer some protection against a pandemic strain and possibly save many lives in the first critical months of an outbreak.

We're also increasing stockpiles of antiviral drugs, such as Tamiflu and Relenza. Antiviral drugs cannot prevent people from contracting the flu, but they can reduce the severity of the illness when taken within 48 hours of getting sick.

So in addition to vaccines, which are the foundation of our pandemic response, I'm asking Congress for $1 billion to stockpile additional antiviral medications so that we have enough on hand to help treat first responders and those on the front lines as well as populations most at risk in the first stages of a pandemic.

To protect the greatest possible number of Americans during a pandemic, the cornerstone of our strategy is to develop new technologies that will allow us to produce new vaccines rapidly.

If a pandemic strikes, our country must have a surge capacity in place that will allow us to bring a new vaccine on-line quickly and manufacture enough to immunize every American against the pandemic strain.

I recently met with leaders of the vaccine industry. They assured me that they will work with the federal government to expand the vaccine industry so that our country is better prepared for any pandemic.

Today, the NIH is working with vaccine makers to develop new cell culture techniques that will help us bring a pandemic flu vaccine to the American people faster in the event of an outbreak.

Right now, most vaccines are still produced with 1950s technology, using chicken eggs that are infected with the influenza virus and then used to develop and produce vaccines.

In the event of a pandemic, this antiquated process would take many, many months to produce a vaccine, and it would not allow us to produce enough vaccine for every American in time.

Since American lives depend on rapid advances in vaccine production technology, we must fund a crash program to help our best scientists bring the next generation of technology on-line rapidly.

I'm asking Congress for $2.8 billion to accelerate development of cell culture technology. By bringing cell culture technology from the research laboratory into the production line, we should be able to produce enough vaccine for every American within six months of the start of a pandemic.

I'm also asking Congress to remove one of the greatest obstacles to domestic vaccine production: the growing burden of litigation.

In the past three decades, the number of vaccine manufacturers in America has plummeted as the industry has been flooded with lawsuits. Today, there's only one manufacturer in the United States that can produce influenza vaccine. That leaves our nation vulnerable in the event of a pandemic.

We must increase the number of vaccine manufacturers in our country and improve our domestic production capacity.

So Congress must pass liability protection for the makers of life-saving vaccines.

By making wise investments in technology and breaking down barriers to vaccine production, we're working toward a clear goal: In the event of a pandemic we must have enough vaccine for every American.

The third part of our strategy is to ensure that we're ready to respond to a pandemic outbreak.

A pandemic is unlike other natural disasters. Outbreaks can happen simultaneously in hundreds, or even thousands, of locations at the same time. And unlike storms or floods which strike in an instant and then recede, a pandemic can continue spreading destruction in repeated ways that can last for a year or more.

To respond to a pandemic we must have emergency plans in place in all 50 states, in every local community. We must ensure that all levels of government are ready to act to contain an outbreak. We must be able to deliver vaccines and other treatments to front-line responders and at-risk populations.

So my administration is working with public health officials in the medical community to develop effective pandemic emergency plans. We're working at the federal level. We're looking at ways and options to coordinate our response with state and local leaders.

I've asked Mike Leavitt -- Secretary Leavitt to bring together state and local public health officials from across the nation to discuss their plans for a pandemic and to help them improve pandemic planning at the community level.

I'm asking Congress to provide $583 million for pandemic preparedness, including $100 million to help states complete and exercise their pandemic plans now before a pandemic strikes.

If an influenza pandemic strikes every nation, every state in this union and every community in these states must be ready.

To respond to a pandemic we need medical personnel and adequate supplies of equipment. In a pandemic, everything from syringes to hospital beds, respirators, masks and protective equipment would be in short supply.

So the federal government is stockpiling critical supplies in locations across America as part of the Strategic National Stockpile.

The Department of Health and Human Services is helping states create rosters of medical personnel who are willing to help alleviate local shortfalls during a pandemic.

And every federal department involved in health care is expanding plans to ensure that all federal medical facilities, personnel and response capabilities are available to support local communities in the event of a pandemic crisis.

To respond to a pandemic, the American people need to have information to protect themselves and others. In a pandemic, an infection carried by one person can be transmitted to many other people, and so every American must take personal responsibility for stopping the spread of the virus.

To provide Americans with more information about pandemics, we are launching a new Web site, pandemicflu.gov. That ought to be easy for people to remember: pandemicflu.gov.

The Web site will keep our citizens informed about the preparations under way, steps they can take now to prepare for a pandemic, and what every American can do to decrease their risk of contracting and spreading the disease in the event of an outbreak.

To respond to a pandemic, members of the international community will continue to work together. An influenza pandemic would be an event with global consequences, and therefore we continue to meet to develop a global response.

We've called nations together in the past, and we'll continue to call nations together, to work with public health experts to better coordinate our efforts to deal with a disaster.

Now, all of the steps I've outlined today require immediate resources. Because a pandemic could strike at any time, we can't waste time in preparing. So to meet all our goals, I'm requesting a total of $7.1 billion in emergency funding from the United States Congress.

By making critical investments today, we'll strengthen our ability to safeguard the American people in the awful event of a devastating global pandemic; and at the same time, we'll bring our nation's public health and medical infrastructure more squarely in the 21st century.

The steps I've outlined will also help our nation in other critical ways.

By perfecting cell-based technologies now, we will be able to produce vaccines for a range of illnesses and save countless lives.

By strengthening our domestic vaccine industry, we can help ensure that our nation will never again have a shortage of vaccine for seasonal flu.

And by putting in place and exercising pandemic emergency plans across the nation, we can help our nation prepare for other dangers, such as a terrorist attack using chemical or biological weapons.

Leaders at every level of government have a responsibility to confront dangers before they appear and engage the American people in the best course of action. It is vital that our nation discuss and address the threat of pandemic flu now.

There is no pandemic flu in our country or in the world at this time. But if we wait for a pandemic to appear, it will be too late to prepare. And one day many lives could be needlessly lost because we failed to act today.

By preparing now, we can give our citizens some peace of mind, knowing that our nation is ready to act at the first sign of danger and that we have the plans in place to prevent and, if necessary, withstand an influenza pandemic.

Thank you for coming today to let me outline my strategy. Thank the United States Congress for considering this measure.

May God bless you all."

CHAPTER THIRTEEN

NATIONAL STRATEGY FOR PANDEMIC INFLUENZA

Introduction

Although remarkable advances have been made in science and medicine during the past century, we are constantly reminded that we live in a universe of microbes - viruses, bacteria, protozoa and fungi that are forever changing and adapting themselves to the human host and the defenses that humans create.

Influenza viruses are notable for their resilience and adaptability. While science has been able to develop highly effective vaccines and treatments for many infectious diseases that threaten public health, acquiring these tools is an ongoing challenge with the influenza virus. Changes in the genetic makeup of the virus require us to develop new vaccines on an annual basis and forecast which strains are likely to predominate.

As a result, and despite annual vaccinations, the U.S. faces a burden of influenza that results in approximately 36,000 deaths and more than 200,000 hospitalizations each year. In addition to this human toll, influenza is annually responsible for a total cost of over $10 billion in the U.S.

A pandemic, or worldwide outbreak of a new influenza virus, could dwarf this impact by overwhelming our health and medical capabilities, potentially resulting in hundreds of thousands of deaths, millions of hospitalizations, and hundreds of billions of dollars in direct and indirect costs. This *Strategy* will guide our preparedness and response activities to mitigate that impact.

The Pandemic Threat

Pandemics happen when a novel influenza virus emerges that infects and can be efficiently transmitted between humans. Animals are the most likely reservoir for these emerging viruses; avian viruses played a role in the last three influenza pandemics. Two of these pandemic-causing viruses remain in circulation and are responsible for the majority of influenza cases each year.

Pandemics have occurred intermittently over centuries. The last three pandemics, in 1918, 1957 and 1968, killed approximately 40 million, 2 million and 1 million people worldwide, respectively. Although the timing cannot be predicted, history and science suggest that we will face one or more pandemics in this century.

The current pandemic threat stems from an unprecedented outbreak of avian influenza in Asia and Europe, caused by the H5N1 strain of the Influenza A virus. To date, the virus has infected birds in 16 countries and has resulted in the deaths, through illness and culling, of approximately 200 million birds across Asia. While traditional control measures have been attempted, the virus is now endemic in Southeast Asia, present in long-range migratory birds, and unlikely to be eradicated soon.

A notable and worrisome feature of the H5N1 virus is its ability to infect a wide range of hosts, including birds and humans. As of the date of this document, the virus is known to have infected 121 people in four countries, resulting in 62 deaths over the past two years. Although the virus has not yet shown an ability to transmit efficiently between humans, as is seen with the annual influenza virus, there is concern that it will acquire this capability through genetic mutation or exchange of genetic material with a human influenza virus.

It is impossible to know whether the currently circulating H5N1 virus will cause a human pandemic. The widespread nature of H5N1 in birds and the likelihood of mutations over time raise our concerns that the virus will become transmissible between humans, with potentially catastrophic consequences. If this does not happen with the current H5N1 strain, history suggests that a different influenza virus will emerge and result in the next pandemic.

The *National Strategy for Pandemic Influenza*

Preparing for a pandemic requires the leveraging of all instruments of national power, and coordinated action by all segments of government and society. Influenza viruses do not respect the distinctions of race, sex, age, profession or nationality, and are not constrained by geographic boundaries. The next pandemic is likely to come in waves, each lasting months, and pass through communities of all size across the nation and world. While a pandemic will not damage power lines, banks or computer networks, it will ultimately threaten all critical infrastructure by removing essential personnel from the workplace for weeks or months.

This makes a pandemic a unique circumstance necessitating a strategy that extends well beyond health and medical boundaries, to include the sustainment of critical infrastructure, private-sector activities, the movement of goods and services across the nation and the globe, and economic and security considerations. The uncertainties associated with influenza viruses require that our *Strategy* be versatile, to ensure that we are prepared for any virus with pandemic potential, as well as the annual burden of influenza that we know we will face.

The *National Strategy for Pandemic Influenza* guides our preparedness and response to an influenza pandemic, with the intent of (1) stopping, slowing or otherwise limiting the spread of a pandemic to the United States; (2) limiting the domestic spread of a pandemic, and mitigating disease, suffering and death; and (3) sustaining infrastructure and mitigating impact to the economy and the functioning of society.

The *Strategy* will provide a framework for future U.S. Government planning efforts that is consistent with *The National Security Strategy* and the *National Strategy for Homeland Security*. It recognizes that preparing for and responding to a pandemic cannot be viewed as a purely federal responsibility, and that the nation must have a system of plans at all levels of government and in all sectors outside of government that can be integrated to address the pandemic threat. It is guided by the following principles:

- The federal government will use all instruments of national power to address the pandemic threat.

- States and communities should have credible pandemic preparedness plans to respond to an outbreak within their jurisdictions.

- The private sector should play an integral role in preparedness before a pandemic begins, and should be part of the national response.

- Individual citizens should be prepared for an influenza pandemic, and be educated about individual responsibility to limit the spread of infection if they or their family members become ill.

- Global partnerships will be leveraged to address the pandemic threat.

Pillars of the *National Strategy*

Our *Strategy* addresses the full spectrum of events that link a farmyard overseas to a living room in America. While the circumstances that connect these environments are very different, our strategic principles remain relevant. The pillars of our *Strategy* are:

- **Preparedness and Communication**: Activities that should be undertaken before a pandemic to ensure preparedness, and the communication of roles and responsibilities to all levels of government, segments of society and individuals.

- **Surveillance and Detection**: Domestic and international systems that provide continuous "situational awareness," to ensure the earliest warning possible to protect the population.

- **Response and Containment**: Actions to limit the spread of the outbreak and to mitigate the health, social and economic impacts of a pandemic.

Implementation of the *National Strategy*

This *Strategy* reflects the federal government's approach to the pandemic threat. While it provides strategic direction for the Departments and Agencies of the U.S. Government, it does not attempt to catalogue and assign all federal responsibilities. The implementation of this *Strategy* and specific responsibilities will be described separately.

Pillar One: Preparedness and Communication

Preparedness is the underpinning of the entire spectrum of activities, including surveillance, detection, containment and response efforts. We will support pandemic planning efforts, and clearly communicate expectations to individuals, communities and governments, whether overseas or in the United States, recognizing that all share the responsibility to limit the spread of infection in order to protect populations beyond their borders.

Planning for a Pandemic

To enhance preparedness, we will:

- Develop federal implementation plans to support this *Strategy*, to include all components of the U.S. government and to address the full range of consequences of a pandemic, including human and animal health, security, transportation, economic, trade and infrastructure considerations.

- Work through multilateral health organizations such as the World Health Organization (WHO), Food and Agriculture Organization (FAO), World Organization for Animal Health (OIE) and regional organizations such as the Asia-Pacific Economic Cooperation (APEC) forum, as well as through bilateral and multilateral contacts to:

  o Support the development and exercising of avian and pandemic response plans;

  o Expand in-country medical, veterinary and scientific capacity to respond to an outbreak; and

  o Educate populations at home and abroad about high-risk practices that increase the likelihood of virus transmission between species.

- Continue to work with states and localities to:

  o Establish and exercise pandemic response plans;

  o Develop medical and veterinary surge capacity plans; and

  o Integrate non-health sectors, including the private sector and critical infrastructure entities, in these planning efforts.

- Build upon existing domestic mechanisms to rapidly recruit and deploy large numbers of health, medical and veterinary providers within or across jurisdictions to match medical requirements with capabilities.

Communicating Expectations and Responsibilities

A critical element of pandemic planning is ensuring that people and entities not accustomed to responding to health crises understand the actions and priorities required to prepare for and respond to a pandemic. Those groups include political leadership at all levels of government, non-health components of government and members of the private sector. Essential planning also includes the coordination of efforts between human and animal health authorities. In order to accomplish this, we will:

- Work to ensure clear, effective and coordinated risk communication, domestically and internationally, before and during a pandemic. This includes identifying credible spokespersons at all levels of government to effectively coordinate and communicate helpful, informative messages in a timely manner.

- Provide guidance to the private sector and critical infrastructure entities on their role in the pandemic response, and considerations necessary to maintain essential services and operations despite significant and sustained worker absenteeism.

- Provide guidance to individuals on infection control behaviors they should adopt pre-pandemic, and the specific actions they will need to take during a severe influenza season or pandemic, such as self-isolation and protection of others if they themselves contract influenza.

- Provide guidance and support to poultry, swine and related industries on their role in responding to an outbreak of avian influenza, including ensuring the protection of animal workers and initiating or strengthening public education campaigns to minimize the risks of infection from animal products.

Producing and Stockpiling Vaccines, Antivirals and Medical Material

In combination with traditional public health measures, vaccines and antiviral drugs form the foundation of our infection control strategy. Vaccination is the most important element of this strategy, but we acknowledge that a two-pronged strategy incorporating both vaccines and antivirals is essential. To establish production capacity and stockpiles in support of our containment and response strategies, we will:

- Encourage nations to develop production capacity and stockpiles to support their response needs, to include pooling of efforts to create regional capacity.

- Encourage and subsidize the development of state-based antiviral stockpiles to support response activities.

- Ensure that our national stockpile and stockpiles based in states and communities are properly configured to respond to the diversity of medical requirements presented by a pandemic, including personal protective equipment, antibiotics and general supplies.

- Establish domestic production capacity and stockpiles of countermeasures to ensure:

    o Sufficient vaccine to vaccinate front-line personnel and at-risk populations, including military personnel;

    o Sufficient vaccine to vaccinate the entire U.S. population within six months of the emergence of a virus with pandemic potential; and

    o Antiviral treatment for those who contract a pandemic strain of influenza.

- Facilitate appropriate coordination of efforts across the vaccine manufacturing sector.

- Address regulatory and other legal barriers to the expansion of our domestic vaccine production capacity.

- Expand the public health recommendations for domestic seasonal influenza vaccination and encourage the same practice internationally.

- Expand the domestic supply of avian influenza vaccine to control a domestic outbreak of avian influenza in bird populations.

Establishing Distribution Plans for Vaccines and Antivirals

It is essential that we prioritize the allocation of countermeasures (vaccines and antivirals) that are in limited supply and define effective distribution modalities during a pandemic. We will:

- Develop credible countermeasure distribution mechanisms for vaccine and antiviral agents prior to and during a pandemic.

- Prioritize countermeasure allocation before an outbreak, and update this prioritization immediately after the outbreak begins based on the at-risk populations, available supplies and the characteristics of the virus.

Advancing Scientific Knowledge and Accelerating Development

Research and development of vaccines, antivirals, adjuvants and diagnostics represents our best defense against a pandemic. To realize our goal of next-generation countermeasures against influenza, we must make significant and targeted investments in promising technologies. We will:

- Ensure that there is maximal sharing of scientific information about influenza viruses between governments, scientific entities and the private sector.

- Work with our international partners to ensure that we are all leveraging the most advanced technological approaches available for vaccine production.

- Accelerate the development of cell culture technology for influenza vaccine production and establish a domestic production base to support vaccination demands.

- Use novel investment strategies to advance the development of next-generation influenza diagnostics and countermeasures, including new antivirals, vaccines, adjuvant technologies, and countermeasures that provide protection across multiple strains and seasons of the influenza virus.

Pillar Two: Surveillance and Detection

Early warning of a pandemic and our ability to closely track the spread of avian influenza outbreak is critical to being able to rapidly employ resources to contain the spread of the virus. An effective surveillance and detection system will save lives by allowing us to activate our response plans before the arrival of a pandemic virus to the U.S., activate additional surveillance systems and initiate vaccine production and administration.

Ensuring Rapid Reporting of Outbreaks

To support our need for "situational awareness," both domestically and internationally, we will:

- Work through the International Partnership on Avian and Pandemic Influenza, as well as through other political and diplomatic channels such as the United Nations and the Asia-Pacific Economic Cooperation forum, to ensure transparency, scientific cooperation and rapid reporting of avian and human influenza cases.

- Support the development of the proper scientific and epidemiologic expertise in affected regions to ensure early recognition of changes in the pattern of avian or human outbreaks.

- Support the development and sustainment of sufficient U.S. and host nation laboratory capacity and diagnostic reagents in affected regions and domestically, to provide rapid confirmation of cases in animals or humans.

- Advance mechanisms for "real-time" clinical surveillance in domestic acute care settings such as emergency departments, intensive care units and laboratories to provide local, state and federal public health officials with continuous awareness of the profile of illness in communities, and leverage all federal medical capabilities, both domestic and international, in support of this objective.

- Develop and deploy rapid diagnostics with greater sensitivity and reproducibility to allow onsite diagnosis of pandemic strains of influenza at home and abroad, in animals and humans, to facilitate early warning, outbreak control and targeting of antiviral therapy.

- Expand our domestic livestock and wildlife surveillance activities to ensure early warning of the spread of an outbreak to our shores.

Using Surveillance to Limit Spread

Although influenza does not respect geographic or political borders, entry to and egress from affected areas represent opportunities to control or at the very least slow the spread of infection. In parallel to our containment measures, we will:

- Develop mechanisms to rapidly share information on travelers who may be carrying or may have been exposed to a pandemic strain of influenza, for the purposes of contact tracing and outbreak investigation.

- Develop and exercise mechanisms to provide active and passive surveillance during an outbreak, both within and beyond our borders.

- Expand and enhance mechanisms for screening and monitoring animals that may harbor viruses with pandemic potential.

- Develop screening and monitoring mechanisms and agreements to appropriately control travel and shipping of potentially infected products to and from affected regions if necessary, and to protect unaffected populations.

Pillar Three: Response and Containment

We recognize that a virus with pandemic potential anywhere represents a risk to populations everywhere. Once health authorities have signaled sustained and efficient human-to-human spread of the virus has occurred, a cascade of response mechanisms will be initiated, from the site of the documented transmission to locations around the globe.

Containing Outbreaks

The most effective way to protect the American population is to contain an outbreak beyond the borders of the U.S. While we work to prevent a pandemic from reaching our shores, we recognize that slowing or limiting the spread of the outbreak is a more realistic outcome and can save many lives. In support of our containment strategy, we will:

- Work through the International Partnership to develop a coalition of strong partners to coordinate actions to limit the spread of a virus with pandemic potential beyond the location where it is first recognized in order to protect U.S. interests abroad.

- Where appropriate, offer and coordinate assistance from the United States and other members of the International Partnership.

- Encourage all levels of government, domestically and globally, to take appropriate and lawful action to contain an outbreak within the borders of their community, province, state or nation.

- Where appropriate, use governmental authorities to limit non-essential movement of people, goods and services into and out of areas where an outbreak occurs.

- Provide guidance to all levels of government on the range of options for infection-control and containment, including those circumstances where social distancing measures, limitations on gatherings, or quarantine authority may be an appropriate public health intervention.

- Emphasize the roles and responsibilities of the individual in preventing the spread of an outbreak, and the risk to others if infection-control practices are not followed.

- Provide guidance for states, localities and industry on best practices to prevent the spread of avian influenza in commercial, domestic and wild birds, and other animals.

Leveraging National Medical and Public Health Surge Capacity

Rather than generating a focal point of casualties, the medical burden of a pandemic is likely to be distributed in communities across the nation for an extended period of time. In order to save lives and limit suffering, we will:

- Implement state and local public health and medical surge plans, and leverage all federal medical facilities, personnel and response capabilities to support the national surge requirement.

- Activate plans to distribute medical countermeasures, including non-medical equipment and other material, from the Strategic National Stockpile and other distribution centers to federal, state and local authorities.

- Address barriers to the flow of public health, medical and veterinary personnel across state and local jurisdictions to meet local shortfalls in public health, medical and veterinary capacity.

- Determine the spectrum of public health, medical and veterinary surge capacity activities that the U.S. military and other government entities may be able to support during a pandemic, contingent upon primary mission requirements, and develop mechanisms to activate them.

Sustaining Infrastructure, Essential Services and the Economy

Movement of essential personnel, goods and services, and maintenance of critical infrastructure are necessary during an event that spans months in any given community. The private sector and critical infrastructure entities must respond in a manner that allows them to maintain the essential elements of their operations for a prolonged period of time, in order to prevent severe disruption of life in our communities. To ensure this, we will:

- Encourage the development of coordination mechanisms across American industries to support the above activities during a pandemic.

- Provide guidance to activate contingency plans to ensure that personnel are protected, that the delivery of essential goods and services is maintained, and that sectors remain functional despite significant and sustained worker absenteeism.

- Determine the spectrum of infrastructure-sustainment activities that the U.S. military and other government entities may be able to support during a pandemic, contingent upon primary mission requirements, and develop mechanisms to activate them.

Ensuring Effective Risk Communication

Effective risk communication is essential to inform the public and mitigate panic. We will:

- Ensure that timely, clear, coordinated messages are delivered to the American public from trained spokespersons at all levels of government and assist the governments of affected nations to do the same.

- Work with state and local governments to develop guidelines to assure the public of the safety of the food supply and mitigate the risk of exposure from wildlife.

Roles and Responsibilities

Because of its unique nature, responsibility for preparedness and response to a pandemic extends across all levels of government and all segments of society. No single entity alone can prevent or mitigate the impact of a pandemic.

The Federal Government

While the Federal government plays a critical role in elements of preparedness and response to a pandemic, the success of these measures is predicated on actions taken at the individual level and in states and communities. Federal responsibilities include the following:

- Advancing international preparedness, surveillance, response and containment activities.

- Supporting the establishment of countermeasure stockpiles and production capacity by:

    o Facilitating the development of sufficient domestic production capacity for vaccines, antivirals, diagnostics and personal protective equipment to support domestic needs, and encouraging the development of production capacity around the world;

    o Advancing the science necessary to produce effective vaccines, therapeutics and diagnostics; and

    o Stockpiling and coordinating the distribution of necessary countermeasures, in concert with states and other entities.

- Ensuring that federal departments and agencies, including federal health care systems, have developed and exercised preparedness and response plans that take into account the potential impact of a pandemic on the federal workforce, and are configured to support state, local and private sector efforts as appropriate.

- Facilitating state and local planning through funding and guidance.

- Providing guidance to the private sector and public on preparedness and response planning, in conjunction with states and communities.

Lead departments have been identified for the medical response (Department of Health and Human Services), veterinary response (Department of Agriculture), international activities (Department of State) and the overall domestic incident management and Federal coordination (Department of Homeland Security). Each department is responsible for coordination of all efforts within its authorized mission, and departments are responsible for developing plans to implement this *Strategy*.

States and Localities

Our communities are on the front lines of a pandemic and will face many challenges in maintaining continuity of society in the face of widespread illness and increased demand on most essential government services. State and local responsibilities include the following:

- Ensuring that all reasonable measures are taken to limit the spread of an outbreak within and beyond the community's borders.

- Establishing comprehensive and credible preparedness and response plans that are exercised on a regular basis.

- Integrating non-health entities in the planning for a pandemic, including law enforcement, utilities, city services and political leadership.

- Establishing state and community-based stockpiles and distribution systems to support a comprehensive pandemic response.

- Identifying key spokespersons for the community, ensuring that they are educated in risk communication, and have coordinated crisis communications plans.

- Providing public education campaigns on pandemic influenza and public and private interventions.

The Private Sector and Critical Infrastructure Entities

The private sector represents an essential pillar of our society because of the essential goods and services that it provides. Moreover, it touches the majority of our population on a daily basis, through an employer-employee or vendor-customer relationship. For these reasons, it is essential that the U.S. private sector be engaged in all preparedness and response activities for a pandemic.

Critical infrastructure entities also must be engaged in planning for a pandemic because of our society's dependence upon their services. Both the private sector and critical infrastructure entities represent essential underpinnings for the functioning of American society. Responsibilities of the U.S. private sector and critical infrastructure entities include the following:

- Establishing an ethic of infection control in the workplace that is reinforced during the annual influenza season, to include, if possible, options for working offsite while ill, systems to reduce infection transmission, and worker education.

- Establishing contingency systems to maintain delivery of essential goods and services during times of significant and sustained worker absenteeism.

- Where possible, establishing mechanisms to allow workers to provide services from home if public health officials advise against non-essential travel outside the home.

- Establishing partnerships with other members of the sector to provide mutual support and maintenance of essential services during a pandemic.

Individuals and Families

The critical role of individuals and families in controlling a pandemic cannot be overstated. Modeling of the transmission of influenza vividly illustrates the impact of one individual's behavior on the spread of disease, by showing that an infection carried by one person can be transmitted to tens or hundreds of others. For this reason, individual action is perhaps the most important element of pandemic preparedness and response.

Education on pandemic preparedness for the population should begin before a pandemic, should be provided by all levels of government and the private sector, and should occur in the context of preventing the transmission of any infection, such as the annual influenza or the common cold. Responsibilities of the individual and families include:

- Taking precautions to prevent the spread of infection to others if an individual or a family member has symptoms of influenza.

- Being prepared to follow public health guidance that may include limitation of attendance at public gatherings and non-essential travel for several days or weeks.

- Keeping supplies of materials at home, as recommended by authorities, to support essential needs of the household for several days if necessary.

International Partners

We rely upon our international partnerships, with the United Nations, international organizations and private non-profit organizations, to amplify our efforts, and will engage them on a multilateral and bilateral basis. Our international effort to contain and mitigate the effects of an outbreak of pandemic influenza is a central component of our overall strategy. In many ways, the character and quality of the U.S. response and that of our international partners may play a determining role in the severity of a pandemic.

The International Partnership on Avian and Pandemic Influenza stands in support of multinational organizations. Members of the Partnership have agreed that the following 10 principles will guide their efforts:

1. International cooperation to protect the lives and health of our people;

2. Timely and sustained high-level global political leadership to combat avian and pandemic influenza;

3. Transparency in reporting of influenza cases in humans and in animals caused by virus strains that have pandemic potential, to increase understanding and preparedness and especially to ensure rapid and timely response to potential outbreaks;

4. Immediate sharing of epidemiological data and samples with the World Health Organization (WHO) and the international community to detect and characterize the nature and evolution of any outbreaks as quickly as possible, by utilizing, where appropriate, existing networks and mechanisms;

5. Rapid reaction to address the first signs of accelerated transmission of H5N1 and other highly pathogenic influenza strains so that appropriate international and national resources can be brought to bear;

6. Prevent and contain an incipient epidemic through capacity building and in-country collaboration with international partners;

7. Work in a manner complementary to and supportive of expanded cooperation with and appropriate support of key multilateral organizations (including the WHO, Food and Agriculture Organization and World Organization for Animal Health);

8. Timely coordination of bilateral and multilateral resource allocations; dedication of domestic resources (human and financial); improvements in public awareness; and development of economic and trade contingency plans;

9. Increased coordination and harmonization of preparedness, prevention, response and containment activities among nations, complementing domestic and regional preparedness initiatives, and encouraging where appropriate the development of strategic regional initiatives; and

10. Actions based on the best available science.

Through the Partnership and other bilateral and multilateral initiatives, we will promote these principles and support the development of an international capacity to prepare, detect and respond to an influenza pandemic.

Note: The source material for this chapter was obtained from the United States White House website.

Printed in the United Kingdom
by Lightning Source UK Ltd.
110018UKS00002B/36